Workbook for

Respiratory Care Anatomy and Physiology: Foundations for Clinical Practice

Third Edition

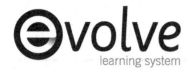
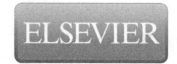
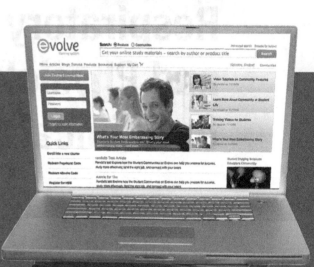

Workbook for

Respiratory Care Anatomy and Physiology: Foundations for Clinical Practice

Third Edition

Will Beachey, PhD, RRT, FAARC
Professor and Director
Respiratory Therapy Program
St. Alexius Medical Center and
The University of Mary
Bismarck, North Dakota

Elizabeth A. Hughes, PhD, RRT, AE-C
Associate Professor
Respiratory Therapy Program
St. Alexius Medical Center and
The University of Mary
Bismarck, North Dakota

Christine K. Sperle, MEd, RRT, AE-C
Assistant Professor and Director of Clinical Education
Respiratory Therapy Program
St. Alexius Medical Center and
The University of Mary
Bismarck, North Dakota

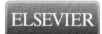

3251 Riverport Lane
St. Louis, Missouri 63043

WORKBOOK FOR RESPIRATORY CARE ANATOMY AND PHYSIOLOGY:
FOUNDATIONS FOR CLINICAL PRACTICE, THIRD EDITION   ISBN: 978-0-323-08586-1

Notices

Knowledge and best practice in this field are constantly changing. As new research and experience broaden our understanding, changes in research methods, professional practices, or medical treatment may become necessary.

Practitioners and researchers must always rely on their own experience and knowledge in evaluating and using any information, methods, compounds, or experiments described herein. In using such information or methods they should be mindful of their own safety and the safety of others, including parties for whom they have a professional responsibility.

With respect to any drug or pharmaceutical products identified, readers are advised to check the most current information provided (i) on procedures featured or (ii) by the manufacturer of each product to be administered, to verify the recommended dose or formula, the method and duration of administration, and contraindications. It is the responsibility of practitioners, relying on their own experience and knowledge of their patients, to make diagnoses, to determine dosages and the best treatment for each individual patient, and to take all appropriate safety precautions.

To the fullest extent of the law, neither the Publisher nor the authors, contributors, or editors, assume any liability for any injury and/or damage to persons or property as a matter of products liability, negligence or otherwise, or from any use or operation of any methods, products, instructions, or ideas contained in the material herein.

Previous editions copyrighted
ISBN: 978-0-8151-2582-2

Content Manager: Billie Sharp
Content Development Specialist: Betsy McCormac
Publishing Services Manager: Julie Eddy
Project Manager: Anita Somaroutu
Designer: Paula Catalano

Printed in the United States of America

Last digit is the print number: 9   8   7   6   5   4   3   2   1

To Jim, Caity, Andrew and Mom, for your support, patience and encouragement.

EAH

To Leon, Aaron, and Jordan for your patience, understanding, and love.

CKS

To Dr. Will Beachey for your ongoing mentorship.

EAH, CKS

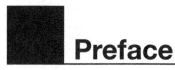

Preface

Respiratory therapists are expected to have a strong foundation in respiratory anatomy and physiology, and this workbook is designed to help the student develop that foundation. Our goal with this workbook is to help the student master information found in Beachey's *Respiratory Care Anatomy and Physiology: Foundations for Clinical Practice*, 3rd edition. A workbook requires active participation in the learning process, something that we believe helps a student to fine-tune their critical thinking skills.

We suggest that students use the workbook as a guide to essential information in the text. Each chapter begins with key terms and definitions that will be very important to understand before moving forward with the concepts presented. Diagrams, short answer questions and critical thinking questions are included in the next section to support what is learned from the textbook. The case studies included in each chapter allow the students to apply what they have learned to the clinical setting, and the key concept questions at the end of each chapter provide a review of important anatomic and physiologic considerations of the cardiopulmonary system. Answers to workbook questions can be found on the Evolve website.

After completing the workbook exercises, students will have gained considerable insight into complex disease processes, and the diagnostic processes and therapeutics required to provide safe, effective respiratory care.

Elizabeth A. Hughes, PhD, RRT, AE-C
Christine K. Sperle, MEd, RRT, AE-C

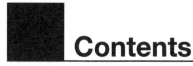

Contents

The Airways and Alveoli

OBJECTIVES

After reading this chapter, you will be able to:

- Differentiate between the structures of upper and lower airways.
- Describe how upper and lower airways differ in their ability to filter, humidify, and warm inspired gas.
- List the goals of artificial airway humidification when natural humidification mechanisms are bypassed.
- Describe what keeps the large cartilaginous airways and small noncartilaginous airways patent.
- Explain why the larger upper airways normally present more resistance to airflow than the smaller lower airways.
- Identify the difference between conducting airways and the respiratory zones of the lung.
- Describe how the various lung clearance mechanisms function and interact.
- List the optimal conditions for effective mucociliary lung clearance.
- Explain the way in which various abnormal physiologic processes impair the effectiveness of lung clearance mechanisms.

KEY TERMS AND DEFINITIONS

Define the following terms:

1. Atelectasis

2. Edema

3. Intubation

4. Tracheostomy

5. Bronchospasm

6. Laryngospasm

7. Intrapulmonary shunt

1

8. Hypoxemia

9. Humidity deficit

10. Ventilator associated pneumonia (VAP)

MATCHING

Match the following terms with the appropriate statement:

_____ 1. Opening to the larynx

_____ 2. Marks the transition between the upper and lower airways

_____ 3. Cartilaginous structure that prevents food from entering the larynx and trachea

_____ 4. Point of division between the right and left mainstem bronchi

_____ 5. Conchae are also called

_____ 6. Passageway that extends from the nasal cavities to the larynx

_____ 7. Mucus-secreting layer of the respiratory tract

_____ 8. Functional respiratory unit of the lung

_____ 9. Space between the alveolar epithelium and capillary endothelium

A. Acinus
B. Carina
C. Epiglottis
D. Glottis
E. Larynx
F. Interstitium
G. Mucosa
H. Pharynx
I. Turbinates

LABELING

1. Label the following structures of the respiratory system:

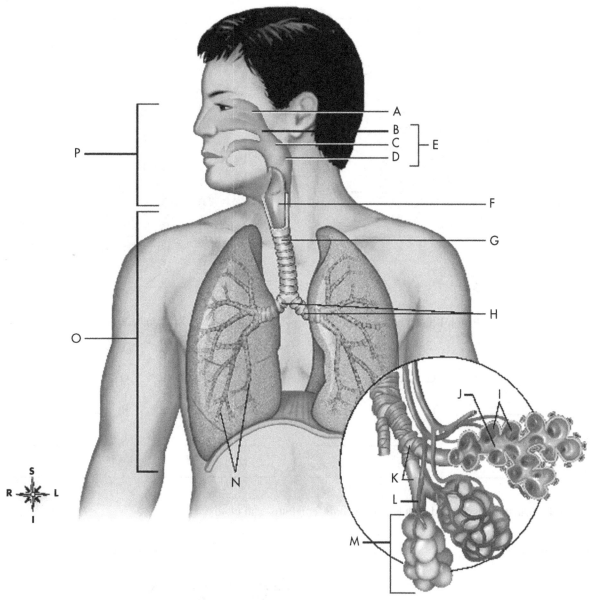

(From Patton KT, Thibodeau GA: *Anatomy & physiology,* ed 7, St. Louis, 2010, Mosby.)

A. _____

B. _____

C. _____

D. _____

E. _____

F. _____

G. _____

H. _____

I. _____

J. _____

K. _____

L. _____

M. _____

N. _____

O. _____

P. _____

2. Label the following structures of the larynx:
   Note: some structures may be shown on both views.

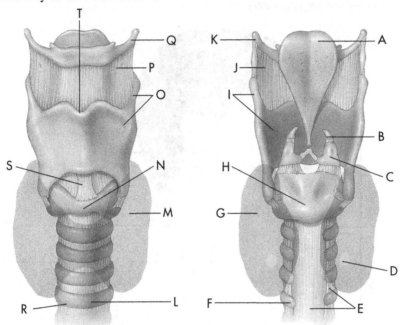

(From Patton KT, Thibodeau GA: *Anatomy & physiology,* ed 7, St. Louis, 2010, Mosby.)

A. _____   F. _____   K. _____   P. _____

B. _____   G. _____   L. _____   Q. _____

C. _____   H. _____   M. _____   R. _____

D. _____   I. _____   N. _____   S. _____

E. _____   J. _____   O. _____   T. _____

3. Label the structures associated with the vocal cords, epiglottis, and glottis:

A. _____

B. _____

C. _____

D. _____

E. _____

F. _____

G. _____

H. _____

I. _____

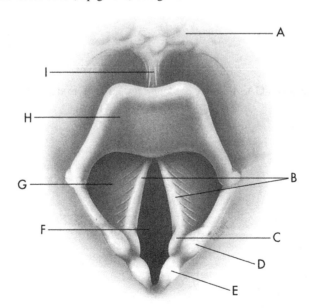

(From Patton KT, Thibodeau GA: *Anatomy & physiology,*
ed 7, St. Louis, 2010, Mosby.)

4. Referring to the diagram below and the textbook, answer the following questions:

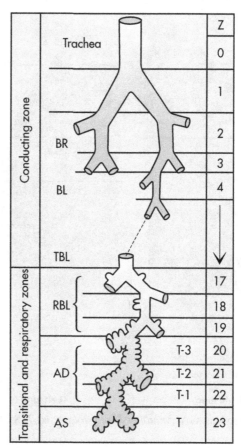

(Modified with permission from Springer Science+Business Media: *Morphometry of the human lung,* 1963, Weibel ER, Berlin, Springer-Verlag. Courtesy Ewald R. Weibel.)

A. Gas exchange between inspired air and circulating blood occurs in which zone? _____

B. At which level do the alveoli first appear? _____

C. Cartilage resembling that found in the trachea is located in level(s) _____.

D. The _____ is the point of division for the mainstem bronchi. The external

landmark for this division point is the _____ thoracic vertebra.

E. Which mainstem bronchus divides more sharply away from the trachea?

5. Label the following structures, lobes, and fissures of the lung.

I.

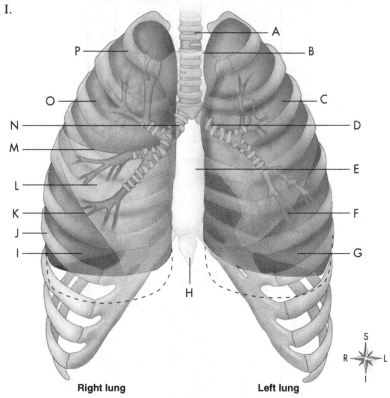

(From Patton KT, Thibodeau GA: *Anatomy & physiology,* ed 7, St. Louis, 2010, Mosby.)

A. _____

B. _____

C. _____

D. _____

E. _____

F. _____

G. _____

H. _____

I. _____

J. _____

K. _____

L. _____

M. _____

N. _____

O. _____

P. _____

II. Label the lobes and segment of the right lung.

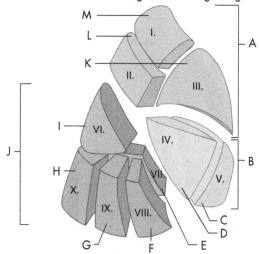

(From Patton KT, Thibodeau GA: *Anatomy & physiology,* ed 7, St. Louis, 2010, Mosby.)

A. _____   F. _____   K. _____

B. _____   G. _____   L. _____

C. _____   H. _____   M. _____

D. _____   I. _____

E. _____   J. _____

III. Label the lobes and segments of the left lung.

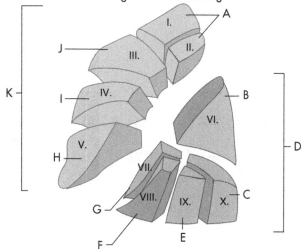

(From Patton KT, Thibodeau GA: *Anatomy & physiology,* ed 7, St. Louis, 2010, Mosby.)

A. _____   E. _____   I. _____

B. _____   F. _____   J. _____

C. _____   G. _____   K. _____

D. _____   H. _____

7

6. Label the following structures of the gas-exchanging portion of the lung:

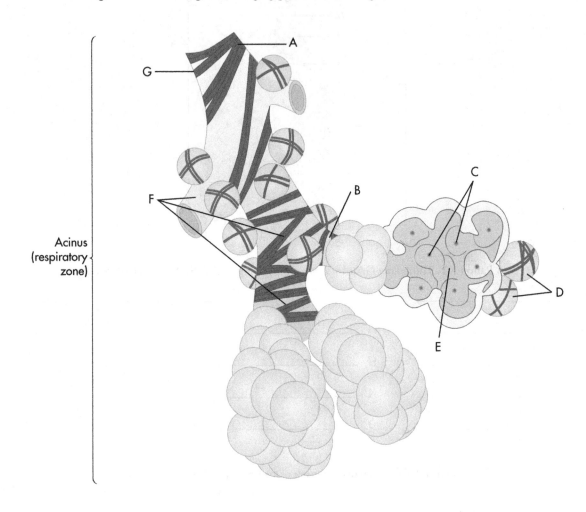

A. _____   E. _____

B. _____   F. _____

C. _____   G. _____

D. _____

7. Label the cellular features of the following cross-sectional diagram:

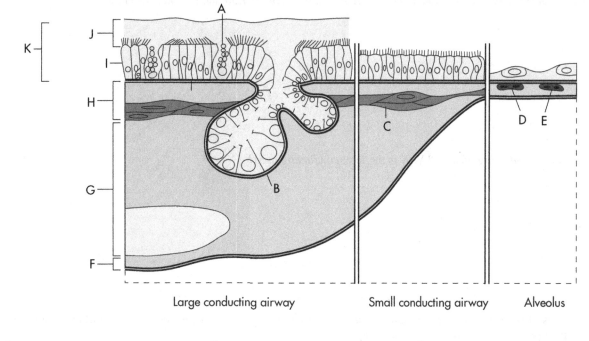

Large conducting airway   Small conducting airway   Alveolus

A. _____   E. _____   I. _____

B. _____   F. _____   J. _____

C. _____   G. _____   K. _____

D. _____   H. _____

8. Referring to the textbook and the figure of the respiratory mucosal epithelium above, answer the following questions:

A. The mucous blanket is formed by secretions from _____ and _____.

B. The mucous blanket is composed of two layers. The upper portion is called the _____ layer;

the function of this layer is _____ _____. The lower portion is called the

_____ layer.

C. Describe how the mucous blanket is propelled up through the airway.

D. Approximately how much mucus is secreted per day in a normal, healthy person?

E. What conditions could decrease the effectiveness of mucociliary clearance?

Chapter **1** **The Airways and Alveoli**

1. Distinguish between *ventilation* and *respiration*, and between *internal* and *external* respiration.

2. What are *conducting airways*? Why is the term *conducting* used?

3. In terms of *filtering, humidifying,* and *warming* the inspired air, what advantage do the nasal turbinates give over a simple open, unobstructed nasal passageway?

4. If a sealed container of air is warmed without adding or subtracting water vapor to the air, what effect does warming it have on the air's capacity for water vapor, and on the air's relative humidity?

5. When room temperature air is inspired into the nasopharynx, what happens to the air temperature, water vapor capacity, water vapor content, and relative humidity? Under what conditions does water evaporate from moist nasal mucous membranes into incoming air?

Chapter **1   The Airways and Alveoli**

6. By what mechanism may artificial airways adversely affect airway humidity and mucus viscosity?

7. What causes *obstructive sleep apnea*?

8. What is the origin of the sound called *stridor*?

9. What is the difference between *croup* and *epiglottitis*?

10. Besides speech, what are other important functions of the vocal cords?

11. Why is the presence of cartilage important in the trachea and large airways?

12. Why does inserting an endotracheal tube too deep into the trachea tend to reduce or prevent ventilation of the left lung?

13. What keeps small, non-cartilaginous airways patent? What is the name for these airways?

14. What percentage of a single breath volume remains in the conducting airways at the end of an inspiration? Why is this important? Would endotracheal intubation change this percentage? Explain.

15. Describe the components of the *acinus*. What structures are present in the acinus that are not present in higher airways? What is the function of these structures?

16. Which general site in the tracheobronchial tree offers the greatest resistance to airflow: all upper airways combined or all lower airways combined? Explain.

17. Describe how mucous glands and ciliary activity are affected by tobacco smoke.

18. T or F: In healthy normal lungs, the lower airways (at the acinus level) are normally sterile (free of microorganisms). Why is this true or not true?

19. The presence of numerous *neutrophils* in airway secretions implies what kind of problem? In what way does this alter secretion characteristics?

20. High blood levels of IgE antibodies imply what kind of respiratory disorder? Explain.

21. Explain the sequence of events that precipitate the symptoms of asthma, beginning with antigen attachment to IgE antibodies.

22. Explain how impaired epithelial secretion of chloride ions into the airway lumen (cystic fibrosis) leads to thickened, dehydrated secretions.

23. Inhaled beta-adrenergic drugs are commonly used in asthma for their immediate airway dilating (bronchodilation) properties. By what mechanism do these drugs also enhance mucus hydration and mobility?

24. Compare and contrast alveolar and conducting airway epithelium.

25. What clearance mechanism removes foreign material and microorganisms from the acinus interstitium and pulmonary interstitium? Define *pulmonary interstitium*.

26. Describe the chain of events whereby exposure to cigarette smoke may eventually lead to loss of elastic lung tissue and development of *emphysema*.

CASE STUDY

You are a respiratory therapist called to the emergency department to assist with airway management of a comatose patient. After assessing the patient, you determine that the patient requires an artificial airway. Immediately after intubating the patient, you use your stethoscope to listen to breath sounds as you manually ventilate the patient.

A. What are you trying to find out?

B. After listening carefully to both sides of the patient's chest while manually ventilating the patient through the endotracheal tube, you hear no breath sounds at all. What is the most likely problem?

C. You re-intubate the patient and this time you hear breath sounds in only one lung. Which lung most likely has the absent breath sounds, and why? What action should you take next to correct the situation?

15

D. What diagnostic procedure would definitively verify proper endotracheal tube placement?

E. Assume your patient is able to breathe spontaneously without mechanical assistance, but is still deeply unconscious. Why might intubation be beneficial for this particular patient? If this patient remains intubated, what preventive actions should the therapist employ?

KEY CONCEPT QUESTIONS

*Instructions: Choose the **single** best answer for each multiple choice question.*

1. An important technique in ventilating a patient during cardiopulmonary resuscitation involves tilting the victim's head back and thrusting the jaw forward. This is done to allow:
   A. Better blood flow to the head
   B. Easier passage of air from the mouth to the lungs
   C. Easier mouth alignment
   D. Reduced chance of damage to the upper airways

2. Cromolyn sodium is a drug inhaled into the airways to inhibit mast cell breakdown. This drug would be most useful in treating:
   A. Cystic fibrosis
   B. Ciliary dyskinesia
   C. Allergic asthma
   D. Emphysema

3. In adult respiratory distress syndrome (ARDS), the permeability of the alveolar-capillary membrane is increased. These patients would probably have:
   A. Higher than normal oxygen levels in the blood
   B. Hyperinflated alveoli
   C. Increased blood flow to the alveoli
   D. Increased fluid in the alveoli

4. Because of damage to the lung parenchyma in ARDS, levels of surfactant in the alveoli are reduced. It is not unusual for ARDS patients to require mechanical ventilation. One would expect the ventilator pressure required to deliver each breath to be:
   A. Higher than normally required
   B. Less than normally required
   C. Equal to that normally required
   D. Unaffected by the presence of ARDS

The Lungs and Chest Wall

OBJECTIVES

After reading this chapter, you will be able to:

- Differentiate between the lobes and segments of the right and left lungs.
- Explain why the pleural membranes normally have a subatmospheric pressure between them, and explain the way in which this subatmospheric pressure is related to lung volume.
- Discuss why the systemic bronchial circulation in the lungs prevents alveolar gas and arterial blood oxygen pressures from being equal.
- Identify why sympathetic, parasympathetic, and nonadrenergic, noncholinergic nerve stimulation cause different effects in the lung.
- List the neuronal effects a drug must have to elicit bronchodilation.
- Describe the essential components of an effective cough and the factors that impair cough effectiveness.
- Identify which spinal cord levels correlate with diaphragmatic muscle function.
- Identify the presence of abnormally high respiratory efforts by inspecting the chest.
- Explain the functional difference between primary and accessory muscles of ventilation.

KEY TERMS AND DEFINITIONS

Define the following terms:

1. Agonist

2. Antagonist

3. Anastomoses

4. Neurotransmitter

5. Ganglion

6. Synapse

7. G protein

8. Shunting

9. Dyspnea

10. Thoracentesis

MATCHING

Match the following terms with the appropriate statement:

_____ 1. Connects the visceral pleura with the diaphragm

_____ 2. Left lung portion that overlaps the heart

_____ 3. The area of the lung through which arteries, veins, and the main bronchus enter

_____ 4. The central portion of the chest cavity

_____ 5. Marks the level of the carina and is adjacent to the second rib

_____ 6. Attached to the lung's surface

_____ 7. Point where the lowest margin of the diaphragm meets the chest wall

_____ 8. Area between the visceral and parietal pleura

_____ 9. Attached to the surface of the chest wall

_____ 10. The major muscle of ventilation

A. Parietal pleura
B. Visceral pleura
C. Lingula
D. Pleural space
E. Costophrenic angle
F. Pulmonary ligament
G. Hilum
H. Diaphragm
I. Angle of Louis
J. Mediastinum

Match the following terms with the description of afferent nerves and responses:

_____ 1. Located in the epithelium of the larynx, trachea, and mainstem bronchi

_____ 2. Origin of most afferent nerves

_____ 3. Located in the parenchyma, conducting airways, and pulmonary vasculature

_____ 4. Located near capillaries and alveoli

_____ 5. Part of the Hering-Breuer reflex

_____ 6. Stretch receptors in conducting airway and smooth muscle

_____ 7. Induced by stimulating large airway irritant receptors

A. Vagus
B. Deep inspiration
C. Slow adapting receptors
D. Rapidly adapting receptors
E. Cough reflex
F. J-receptors
G. C-fiber receptors

1. Label the lobes and segments of the right and left lung:

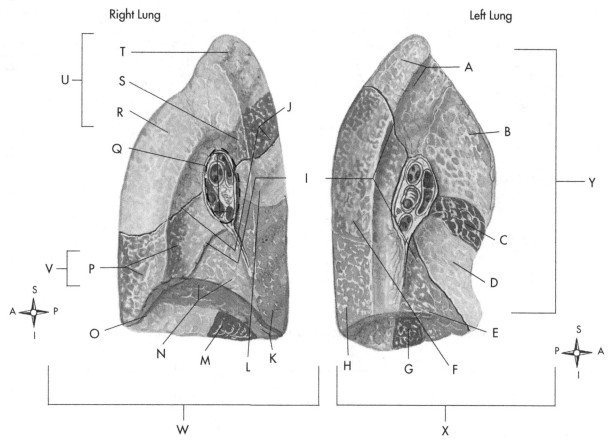

Right Lung   Left Lung

(From Thibodeau GA, Patton KT: *Anatomy & physiology,* ed 3, St Louis, 1996, Mosby.)

A. _____   H. _____   O. _____   V. _____

B. _____   I. _____   P. _____   W. _____

C. _____   J. _____   Q. _____   X. _____

D. _____   K. _____   R. _____   Y. _____

E. _____   L. _____   S. _____

F. _____   M. _____   T. _____

G. _____   N. _____   U. _____

2. Label the neurotransmitters and receptors at the preganglionic and postganglionic neurons for the sympathetic and parasympathetic nervous systems:

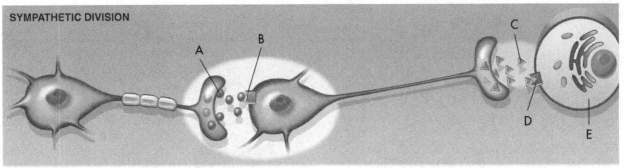

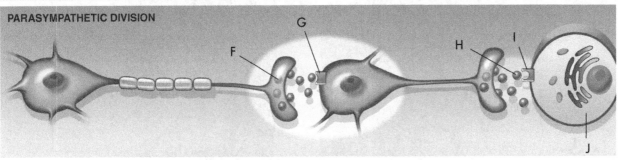

(From Thibodeau GA, Patton KT: *Anatomy & physiology,* ed 5, St Louis, 2003, Mosby.)

A. _____   E. _____   I. _____

B. _____   F. _____   J. _____

C. _____   G. _____

D. _____   H. _____

3. Referring to Table 2-3 in the textbook and the figure above, answer the following questions:

   A. There are different types and subtypes of adrenergic receptors. What are they, and where are they located?

   B. What are the three cholinergic receptors that are present in the human lung? Explain the response that occurs when each receptor is stimulated.

4. Label the following parts of the thoracic cavity:

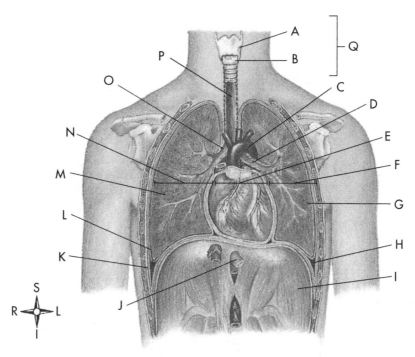

(From Thibodeau GA, Patton KT: *Anatomy & physiology,* ed 3, St Louis, 1996, Mosby.)

A. _____   G. _____   M. _____

B. _____   H. _____   N. _____

C. _____   I. _____   O. _____

D. _____   J. _____   P. _____

E. _____   K. _____   Q. _____

F. _____   L. _____

5. Label the structures of the thoracic cage:

A. _____

B. _____

C. _____

D. _____

E. _____

F. _____

G. _____

H. _____

I. _____

J. _____

K. _____

L. _____

M. _____

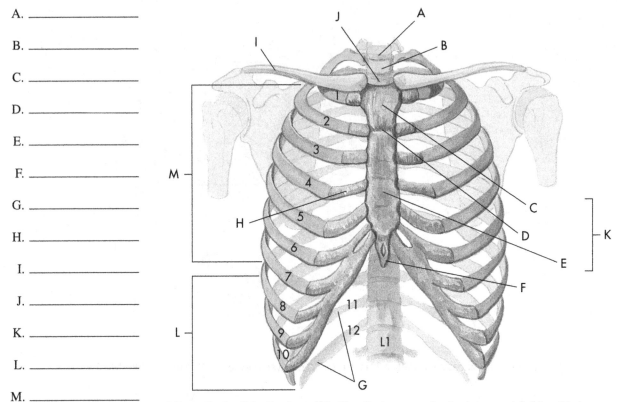

(From Seeley RR, Stephens TD, Tate P: *Anatomy & physiology,* ed 3, New York, 1995, McGraw-Hill.)

6. Label the components of the diaphragm:

A. _____

B. _____

C. _____

D. _____

E. _____

F. _____

G. _____

H. _____

I. _____

J. _____

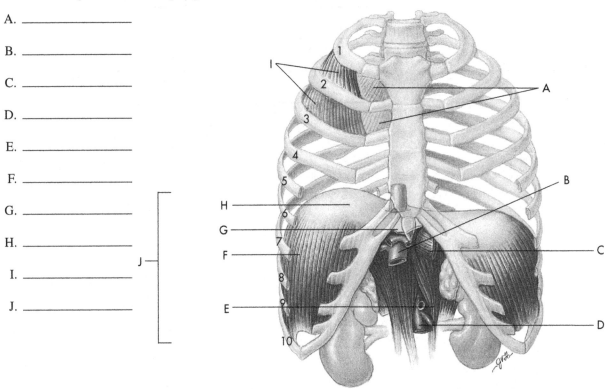

(From Seeley RR, Stephens TD, Tate P: *Anatomy & physiology,* ed 3, New York, 1995, McGraw-Hill.)

7. Label the muscles of ventilation:

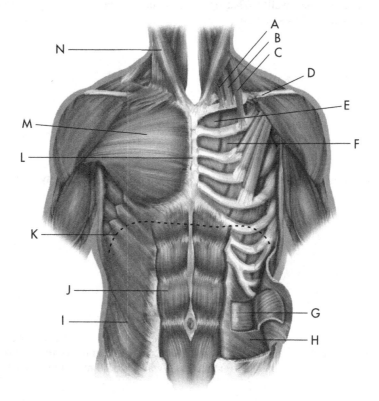

(From Wilkins RL, Stoller JK, Scanlan CL: *Egan's fundamentals of respiratory care,* ed 8, St Louis, 2003, Mosby.)

A. _____   F. _____   K. _____

B. _____   G. _____   L. _____

C. _____   H. _____   M. _____

D. _____   I. _____   N. _____

E. _____   J. _____

SHORT ANSWER/CRITICAL THINKING QUESTIONS

1. The presence of a *pleural effusion* means excessive fluid has collected between the _____ and

   the _____. What would this look like on a chest x-ray image? What would the treatment be for
   this situation?

2. What events would occur if the normal pleural space were made to communicate with atmospheric air (e.g. a puncture wound through the chest wall)? What signs and symptoms might a patient exhibit in this situation? What would be the treatment for this situation?

3. Explain why a pneumothorax will cause the trachea to shift its position—which way might it shift, and why?

4. Considering deoxygenated blood flows from the right ventricle through the lung capillaries where it is exposed to alveolar gas, then leaves the lungs to become arterial blood, what accounts for the difference between the PO_2 of alveolar gas and arterial blood? (i.e. alveolar gas PO_2 is always 5 to 10 mm Hg greater.)

5. What is the likely consequence of a C2 spinal cord transaction?

6. Sympathetic nerve fibers do not innervate the airways; why then does airway smooth muscle respond when the body receives sympathetic stimuli?

7. Vagal stimuli are also known as _____ stimuli, which cause what kind of response in bronchial smooth muscle?

8. During breathing, the "bucket-handle" rib movements mainly change the _____ dimensions of the chest wall.

9. Explain the active and passive diaphragm movements during quiet breathing.

10. Which diaphragmatic fibers have no rib cage attachments? How does their function differ from fibers that have direct rib cage attachments?

11. Under what circumstances does expiration require active muscle contraction in healthy people? Which muscles are involved?

CASE STUDY

A 70-year-old male presents to the emergency department with the complaint of shortness of breath. He is breathing shallowly with a respiratory rate of 30 breaths per minute. His shoulders seem to be fixed in an elevated state and his neck muscles are active. A chest x-ray reveals hyperinflation and flattened diaphragm.

1. Based on these initial findings, what do you suspect is the diagnosis of this patient?

2. Auscultation of the chest reveals diminished breath sounds with faint expiratory wheezes throughout all lung fields, indicating the need for inhaled bronchodilator therapy. What type of drug do you suggest be used for this patient, and how did you come to this conclusion?

3. Some patients with increased airway resistance benefit from the combination of a beta$_2$-agonist bronchodilator and an anticholinergic bronchodilator. What do you think would be the benefit of using a combination drug in this particular patient?

KEY CONCEPT QUESTIONS

*Instructions: Choose the **single** best answer for each multiple choice question.*

1. Fluid removal and filtering in interstitial spaces (spaces between cells and vessels) is accomplished in the lung by the:
   A. Pulmonary circulation
   B. Lymphatic system
   C. Bronchial circulation
   D. Mucociliary clearance mechanism

2. Comatose patients often lose irritant receptor response. As a result, these patients would probably be at increased risk for:
   A. Pleural effusion
   B. Bronchoconstriction
   C. Excessive coughing
   D. Aspiration of foreign material

3. An obese individual with a large abdomen may exhibit a shallow respiratory pattern (small tidal volumes) at rest. What would be the most likely reason?
   A. Elastic recoil of the lung is limited in obese individuals
   B. Diaphragmatic movement is limited in obese individuals
   C. Increased physical exertion is present even at rest
   D. Abnormal respiratory musculature is present

4. A patient with advanced, severe chronic obstructive pulmonary disease (COPD) is leaning forward on a bedside table, grasping its edges while breathing at rest. Scalene and sternomastoid muscle activity is visible. These observations indicate:
   A. Probable nerve damage to the diaphragm
   B. A normal respiratory pattern
   C. Increased work of breathing
   D. Decreased work of breathing

3 Mechanics of Ventilation

OBJECTIVES

After reading this chapter, you will be able to:

- Explain how elastic recoil forces of the lungs and chest wall interact to establish the resting lung volume.
- Describe how the static lung volumes and capacities are influenced by changes in the elastic recoil forces of the lungs and chest wall.
- Explain which pressure gradients maintain alveolar volume and create airflow into and out of the lung.
- Describe how spontaneous breathing and positive pressure mechanical ventilation are different and similar in the way they create pressure gradients throughout the respiratory cycle.
- Identify how the rib cage, diaphragm, and abdomen components of the thorax move and interact differently in normal and abnormal conditions.
- Derive meaning from the static and dynamic pressure-volume curves of the lungs, thorax, and the lung-thorax system.
- Identify whether high inflation pressure during mechanical ventilation is caused by a change in lung compliance or in airway resistance.
- List what factors cause lung compliance and airway resistance to change.
- Describe how surface tension and pulmonary surfactant influence lung compliance, inflation pressure, alveolar stability, and work of breathing.
- Explain what causes the lung's pressure-volume curve to exhibit hysteresis.
- Explain how to use pressure-volume and time-pressure curves to distinguish between elastic and frictional forces that oppose lung inflation.
- Identify why greater muscular effort fails to increase expiratory flow rates under certain physical conditions.
- Explain how compliance and resistance are related to the emptying and filling rates of the lung during breathing.
- Describe what factors predispose to incomplete exhalation and trapping of positive pressure in the alveoli at the end of expiration.
- Assess and quantify the work of breathing, respiratory muscular strength, and respiratory muscular fatigue.

KEY TERMS AND DEFINITIONS

Define and give the abbreviation for each of the following terms:

1. Intrapleural pressure

2. Alveolar pressure

3. Airway opening pressure

4. Transpulmonary pressure

5. Transthoracic pressure

6. Transrespiratory pressure

7. Body-surface pressure

8. Transairway pressure

9. Equal pressure point

10. Total lung capacity

11. Residual volume

12. Expiratory reserve volume

13. Tidal volume

14. Inspiratory reserve volume

15. Inspiratory capacity

16. Vital capacity

17. Functional residual capacity

18. Maximum inspiratory pressure

19. Maximum expiratory pressure

20. Lower inflection point

21. Upper inflection point

22. Positive end-expiratory pressure

23. Lung compliance

24. Airway resistance

25. Dynamic compliance

26. Static compliance

27. Peak pressure

28. Plateau pressure

29. Peak inspiratory pressure

30. Time constant

MATCHING

1. Match the following descriptors with the appropriate terms for the lung–chest wall mechanics:

_____ 1. Recoil force

_____ 2. Contributes most to lung elasticity

_____ 3. Mouth pressure during spontaneous breathing

_____ 4. Alveolar pressure

_____ 5. Pressure between chest wall and lung

_____ 6. Difference between two pressures

_____ 7. No air flow

_____ 8. Airway opening pressure minus alveolar pressure

_____ 9. Alveolar minus pleural pressure

_____ 10. Alveolar minus body surface pressure

A. Atmospheric pressure
B. Intrapulmonary pressure
C. Pressure gradient
D. Elasticity
E. Transpulmonary pressure
F. Surface tension
G. Transairway pressure
H. Transthoracic pressure
I. Intrapleural pressure
J. Zero pressure gradient

2. Match the following terms with the appropriate descriptors for lung volumes and capacities:

_____ 1. Capacity

_____ 2. Volume

_____ 3. Total lung capacity

_____ 4. Residual volume

_____ 5. Vital capacity

_____ 6. Inspiratory capacity

_____ 7. Expiratory reserve volume

_____ 8. Functional residual capacity

_____ 9. Tidal volume

A. Maximum amount of air exhaled in a single breath after a maximal inspiration
B. Comprised of at least two volumes
C. Maximum inspiratory lung volume from end-tidal level
D. Normal breath
E. Exhalable volume beyond resting end-tidal level
F. Cannot be exhaled
G. Volume remaining in the lung at end-tidal exhalation
H. Subdivision of a capacity
I. Sum of all volumes

3. Match the following terms about dynamic lung–chest wall mechanics with the appropriate descriptors:

_____ 1. Driving pressure

_____ 2. Viscosity

_____ 3. Laminar flow

_____ 4. Turbulent flow

_____ 5. Poiseuille's law

_____ 6. Transitional flow

A. Frictional resistance between gas molecules
B. Pressure gradient
C. High-velocity gas molecules impact airway walls frequently
D. Pressure increases exponentially when airway radius decreases
E. Flow occurring where airways branch
F. Overlapping cylindrical gas layers moving at different speeds

LABELING

Label the pressure gradients involved in ventilation:

1. _____

2. _____

3. _____

4. _____

5. _____

6. _____

7. _____

1. When the respiratory muscles are relaxed and no air is flowing, circle the statement(s) that is/are true? *(E and F fill in the blanks.)*

    A. You are at end-tidal exhalation.

    B. You are at end-tidal inhalation.

    C. You are at the midpoint of tidal inhalation.

    D. The volume of gas in your lung is 0 mL.

    E. The volume of gas in your lung is called the _____

    F. The volume of gas in your lung is determined by which physical forces? _____

2. T or F. If alveolar pressure (P_A) rises, alveolar volume must also rise.

3. T or F. Transrespiratory pressures [($P_A - P_{ao}$) or P_{rs}] are identical at end-inspiration and end-expiration.

4. T or F. Transpulmonary pressures are identical at end-inspiration and end-expiration.

5. If P_A is 763 mm Hg and P_{ao} is 760 mm Hg, the person is at what point in the respiratory cycle?

6. During positive pressure mechanical ventilation, inspired volume is 500 mL. The same person, moments later, spontaneously inspires 500 mL. Compare the following: alveolar pressures; alveolar volumes; transpulmonary pressures; degree of alveolar epithelial stretch.

7. Loss of elastic recoil forces results in **[increased/decreased]** _____ volume and

    _____ capacity.

8. For each cm H_2O pressure, about how much volume can be forced into the normally compliant lung-thorax system at the FRC level? _____

9. In addition to elastic lung fibers, _____ also contributes to the lungs' recoil force.

10. Lungs lacking pulmonary surfactant exhibit **[low/high]** compliance or **[low/high]** recoil force.

11. To exhale the vital capacity (VC), one must first _____ and then exhale until only

    the _____ is left in the lungs. Exhaling the VC in this manner is a **[passive, non-energy-expending/active energy-expending]** process.

12. Why may a person with high airway resistance have a low vital capacity? Why may a person with low lung compliance also have a low vital capacity?

13. Which affects airway resistance the most: airway diameter or airway length?

14. Where is airflow most turbulent: in upper large airways or in lower small airways? Explain.

15. Multiplying compliance by resistance yields a value called the _____

    _____. The unit in which this value is expressed is _____.
    What is the relevance of this value to lung ventilation?

16. Explain why the lungs have a maximum achievable expiratory flow rate at a given lung volume, regardless of how much muscular effort is applied.

CASE STUDIES

1. A 30-year-old female with an exacerbation of asthma is receiving mechanical ventilation. During a routine check of ventilator-patient parameters, you note that over the past 2 hours, peak inspiratory pressures have increased from 24 cm H_2O to 40 cm H_2O and plateau pressures have remained the same at 20 cm H_2O. It has been 2 hours since the patient has received bronchodilator therapy and suctioning.

    A. Based on these findings, what do you suspect is occurring? Explain.

    B. What physical findings would assist you in determining what steps you need to take to treat the patient at this time? Explain.

2. Immediately after birth, a premature infant shows signs of respiratory distress and requires mechanical ventilation. The chest x-ray shows ground glass appearance throughout all lung fields. Lab analysis reveals an L/S ratio of 1:1. High pressures are needed to ventilate the infant.

    A. Based on these findings what do you suspect is occurring? Explain.

    B. What treatment is recommended at this time? Explain.

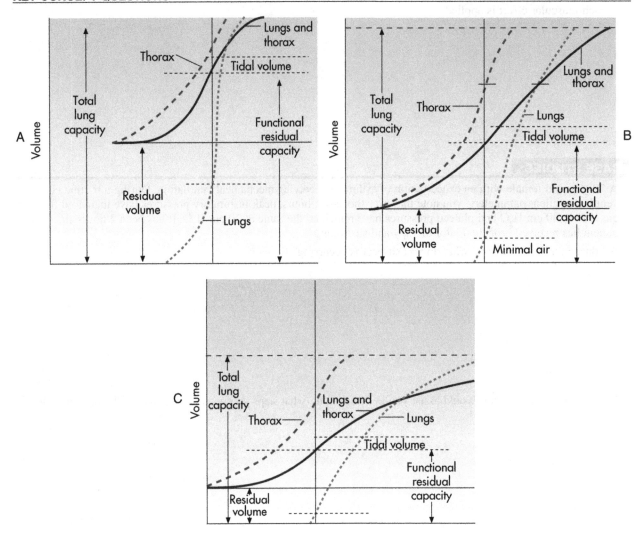

1. Refer to the diagrams above and indicate which diagram (A, B, or C) describes each statement best.

_____ Total compliance is decreased.

_____ Total compliance is increased.

_____ Residual volume percentage of total lung capacity is increased.

_____ Lung compliance is normal.

_____ Lung compliance is increased.

_____ Lung compliance is consistent with chronic obstructive pulmonary disease.

_____ Lung compliance is consistent with fibrotic lung disease.

_____ High lung recoil force is present.

_____ Low lung recoil force is present.

*Instructions: Choose the **single** best answer for each multiple choice question.*

2. Some mechanical ventilators are volume limited. Breath-to-breath volumes delivered to the patient are essentially identical. If a patient's lung compliance decreases, the inspiratory positive pressure required to deliver a mechanical breath would be:
   A. Decreased
   B. Unchanged
   C. Increased
   D. Unrelated to compliance changes

3. An essential component of the cough effort is the ability to increase lung volumes prior to forceful expulsion of inspired air. Patients with obstructive airways disease often have a large total lung capacity, yet they experience difficulty expectorating secretions. The reasons for this include:
   A. Premature airway collapse during forceful expiration
   B. A reduction in functional residual capacity
   C. Increased lung elastic recoil
   D. A reduced equilibrium point for the functional residual capacity

4. According to Poiseuille's law, if a bronchogenic tumor compressed a mainstem bronchus to one half its original diameter, the pressure required to maintain normal ventilation in the affected lung would:
   A. Be unchanged
   B. Double
   C. Be multiplied eight times
   D. Be multiplied sixteen times

4 Ventilation

OBJECTIVES

After reading this chapter, you will be able to:

- Calculate the partial pressures of gases under dry and 100% relative humidity conditions.
- Explain how minute ventilation, alveolar ventilation, and dead space ventilation are interrelated.
- Identify whether hyperventilation or hypoventilation is present by reviewing the arterial carbon dioxide pressure (PCO_2).
- Identify why alveolar ventilation affects arterial PCO_2.
- Identify the rationale underlying the calculation of anatomical dead space, alveolar ventilation, and physiologic and anatomic dead space volume to tidal volume ratios.
- Predict the effects of minute ventilation changes on alveolar ventilation, dead space ventilation, and arterial PCO_2.
- Explain how ventilatory pattern affects dead space volume to tidal volume ratio and, subsequently, alveolar ventilation and arterial PCO_2.
- Describe the theoretical basis for measuring and calculating dead space and alveolar ventilation.

KEY TERMS AND DEFINITIONS

Define the following abbreviations/terms:

1. V_T

2. P_B

3. $\dot{V}_E$

4. $\dot{V}_A$

5. $\dot{V}_D$

6. V_{Danat}

7. V_{DA}

8. $\dot{V}CO_2$

9. V_D/V_T

10. $P_{\bar{E}}CO_2$

11. Hypoventilation

12. Hyperventilation

13. Capnometer

14. Conducting airways

MATCHING

Match the following terms with the appropriate statement:

_____ 1. Nitrogen

_____ 2. Oxygen

_____ 3. Carbon dioxide

_____ 4. Barometric pressure

_____ 5. Dalton's law

_____ 6. Water vapor

A. Trace gas in air
B. 760 mm Hg at sea level
C. Greatest atmospheric partial pressure
D. Pressure must be subtracted to calculate partial pressures in the lung
E. Each gas exerts a partial pressure proportional to its concentration
F. Comprises about 21% of atmospheric air

1. Explain why the PO_2 of inspired room air gas measured in the trachea is less than the PO_2 of room air measured at the mouth? Illustrate by calculating the PO_2 of a gas at room temperature and the PO_2 of a gas at the tracheal level.

2. Your comatose patient is being mechanically ventilated by a machine with these ventilatory controls (each can be independently adjusted):
   Tidal Volume (V_T)
   Respiratory Rate (f)
   The V_T control is set at 500 mL, and the f control is set at 8/min. The $PaCO_2$ is 50 mm Hg. The P_ECO_2 is 33 mm Hg. Calculate the $\dot{V}_E$, the $\dot{V}_A$, and the $\dot{V}_D$.

   A. In an effort to lower the $PaCO_2$, your colleague increases the f to 16/min. Will this decrease the $PaCO_2$?

   B. What is this patient's V_D/V_T now? What is the patient's $PaCO_2$ now? (Hint: recall that V_A and $PaCO_2$ are inversely related, i.e. $\dot{V}_A1 \times PaCO_21 = \dot{V}_A2 \times PaCO_22$, where 1 and 2 refer to initial and final conditions.)

3. A spontaneously breathing patient has a normal $PaCO_2$ of 40 mm Hg, a minute ventilation of 6 L/min, and a V_D/V_T ratio of .35. Then the patient develops a pulmonary embolus, blocking blood flow to a significant number of ventilated alveoli. Consequently, the measured V_D/V_T increases to .65.
   A. Calculate the alveolar ventilation associated with the original $PaCO_2$ of 40 mm Hg.

   B. To maintain the same $PaCO_2$ of 40 after the embolus occurs, what change must occur in total *minute ventilation*?

1. You are caring for a patient on mechanical ventilation that requires bronchodilator therapy. You need to add a small volume nebulizer to the ventilator circuit. You decide to attach a 6-inch length of tubing to the t-piece of the nebulizer and insert it between the endotracheal tube and the Y connector of the inspiratory and expiratory limbs of the ventilator tubing. After the bronchodilator treatment, you decide to leave the nebulizer in place. Several hours later, a routine blood gas is drawn and shows an increase in $PaCO_2$ from a previous blood gas.

   A. What is the most likely cause of the increased $PaCO_2$? Explain.

   B. What would you do to remedy the situation?

2. Patient A has a dead space volume of 150 mL, a tidal volume of 450 mL, and a respiratory frequency of 10. Patient B has a dead space volume of 150 mL, a tidal volume of 350 mL, and a respiratory frequency of 12.

   A. Which patient has the most efficient ventilation?

   B. Why?

*Instructions: Choose the **single** best answer for each multiple choice question.*

1. Patient A has normal conducting airways. Patient B breathes through a tracheostomy tube. The patients have identical breathing rates and tidal volumes and are of similar height and weight. Comparing these two patients, alveolar ventilation is:
   A. Greater in Patient B
   B. Greater in Patient A
   C. The same in both patients
   D. Not comparable for the two patients with the given information

2. If the inspired air in a dehydrated patient's lung is drier than normal, oxygen tension is:
   A. Lower than normal
   B. Higher than atmospheric partial pressure of oxygen
   C. Higher than normal
   D. Equal to the atmospheric partial pressure of oxygen

3. A carbon dioxide monitor attached to the endotracheal tube of an intubated patient reveals an end-tidal carbon dioxide partial pressure that is 3 mm Hg lower than arterial carbon dioxide analyzed at the same time.
   This variance:
   A. Is abnormal; end-tidal PCO_2 should be higher and arterial PCO_2
   B. Represents a normal alveolar-arterial PCO_2 gradient
   C. Represents abnormal alveolar dead space
   D. Is abnormal; the alveolar-arterial PCO_2 gradient is normally greater than 10 mm Hg

4. A bronchodilator drug is administered to a patient experiencing acute, severe airway constriction and hypercapnia. The drug decreases the abnormally high arterial carbon dioxide levels because:
   A. Minute ventilation increases
   B. Alveolar ventilation increases
   C. Tidal volume increases
   D. Dead space volume decreases

5 Pulmonary Function Measurements

OBJECTIVES

After reading this chapter, you will be able to:

- Explain how the normal range of human pulmonary function values are obtained.
- Identify why dilution or washout measurements of functional residual capacity in severe obstructive airway disease generally differ from those obtained by the plethysmographic method.
- Explain why both restrictive and obstructive disease mechanisms reduce the vital capacity.
- Identify why restrictive and obstructive diseases affect the functional residual capacity, the residual volume, and the work of breathing differently.
- Differentiate between purely obstructive and restrictive patterns of pulmonary function tests.
- Explain why large and small airways resistance affects certain spirometric tests in different ways.
- Identify why the results of some spirometric tests can be improved with greater effort, but the results of others are independent of effort.
- Explain the theory behind the test that detects grossly uneven ventilation of the lungs.
- Identify why individuals with severe obstructive pulmonary disease and normal healthy people differ in the relationship between maximum voluntary ventilation and ventilation attained during maximal exercise.
- Explain the basic theory behind tests that are especially sensitive to increases in small airways resistance.

KEY TERMS AND DEFINITIONS

Define the following terms:

1. Anthropometric

2. Closing capacity

3. $FEF_{25\%-75\%}$

4. FEV_1

5. FVC

6. Flow-volume loop

7. Forced expired flow

8. Maximum sustainable ventilation

9. Peak expiratory flow

10. Pneumotachometer

MATCHING

Match the following terms with the appropriate statement:

_____ 1. The greatest amount of air a person can move in and out of their lungs in 10 to 15 seconds

_____ 2. The flow rate at 75% of the forced vital capacity

_____ 3. Pulmonary function tests are reported under these conditions

_____ 4. Test that demonstrates volume left in the lungs when basal small airways close

_____ 5. The volume left in the lung after a complete exhalation, divided by the total lung capacity

_____ 6. The volume exhaled in 1 second during an FVC maneuver.

_____ 7. The volume at which small airways close, regardless of gas density (during a low-density gas spirometry test)

_____ 8. Pulmonary function tests are recorded under these conditions

_____ 9. Highest flow rate generated during an inspiratory forced vital capacity maneuver.

_____ 10. Value representing the volume of air exhaled in 3 seconds during FVC maneuver

A. Ambient temperature, pressure, and saturated (ATPS)
B. Body temperature, pressure, and saturated (BTPS)
C. Closing volume
D. $FEF_{75\%}$
E. FEV_3
F. FEV_1
G. Maximum voluntary ventilation (MVV)
H. Peak inspiratory flow (PIF)
I. RV/TLC ratio
J. Volume of isoflow ($V_{iso}\dot{V}$)

1. On the figure below, label the lung volume or capacity represented by letters A through H, and state the average normal values for each.

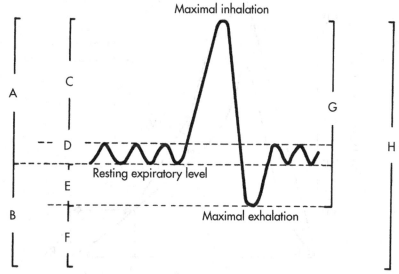

(From Wilkins RL, Stoller JK, Scanlan CL: *Egan's fundamentals of respiratory care,* ed 6, St Louis, 2003, Mosby.)

Lung volume	Average normal value
A. _____	_____
B. _____	_____
C. _____	_____
D. _____	_____
E. _____	_____
F. _____	_____
G. _____	_____
H. _____	_____

2. Label the flow-volume curves (A-C) in the figures below as "normal," "restrictive," or "obstructive."

A. _____

B. _____

C. _____

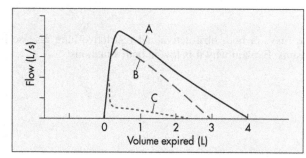

(Redrawn from Fishman AP: *Assessment of pulmonary function,* New York, 1980, McGraw-Hill.)

3. On the graph below, indicate the point of volume isoflow ($V_{iso}\dot{V}$)

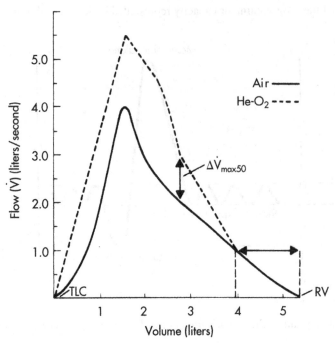

(From Ruppel G: *Manual of pulmonary function testing,* ed 9, St Louis, 2009, Mosby.)

SHORT ANSWER/CRITICAL THINKING QUESTIONS

1. What do the terms *obstructive* and *restrictive* mean with regard to abnormal lung function?

2. What are the main pulmonary function findings in obstructive and restrictive lung diseases?

3. The FEV_1 in both obstructive and restrictive lung disease is generally lower than normal, but for two different reasons. Explain why it is low in both situations.

4. Patient A has an FVC equal to 80% of her predicted value, and an FEV_1/FVC of 0.45. Patient B has an FVC of 50% of her predicted value and an FEV_1/FVC of .85. Which patient has a pulmonary function indicative of obstructive lung disease, and which patient has a restrictive pattern?

5. In an asthmatic patient, which value would you expect to change the most in response to an inhaled beta$_2$-adrenergic (bronchodilator) drug: FVC or FEV_1/FVC? Why?

6. A patient is seen in the clinic after reporting a reduced peak expiratory flow (PEF or PF) reading on her home peak flow meter. In the pulmonary function lab, you document that her PEF has decreased to 50% of her predicted value, and her $FEF_{25\%-75\%}$ has also reduced to less than 50% of her predicted value. What are possible causes of this patient's abnormal pulmonary function test? What is the site of airflow resistance for the PEF? What is the site of airflow resistance for the $FEF_{25\%-75\%}$?

7. You measure a forced vital capacity (FVC) and a slow vital capacity (SVC) from a patient with obstructive lung disease and find that the SVC test demonstrates larger lung volumes than the FVC. Explain.

8. Two of the three indirect methods of lung measurement (helium dilution and nitrogen washout) yield less accurate results in patients with obstructive lung disease than the third method, body plethysmography. Explain.

9. You review the chart of a patient with Guillain-Barré syndrome and find that the pulmonary function test shows a restrictive pattern, even though the physician noted that this patient has no history of lung disease. What is the cause of the restrictive findings in this patient, if lung disease is not present?

10. A patient asks you to help him understand the results of a pulmonary function test he recently completed at a community health fair. He tells you that he does not understand why his pulmonary function values are so different from his wife's values, given that they are the same age and both non-smokers. What do you tell him?

CASE STUDIES

1. You are a respiratory therapist working as a patient educator in an outpatient clinic. You receive a request from one of the family practice physicians to review a patient's spirometry results with her. The patient has just been diagnosed with pulmonary disease and needs to understand what her disease "is all about." She is a long-term smoker who has become progressively short of breath with exertion over the past two years. The recent spirometry test revealed subnormal values for FVC and FEV_1 resulting in an FEV_1/FVC of 50% of predicted. The patient performed spirometry testing before and after receiving a bronchodilator treatment; however, changes in FVC, FEV_1 and FEV_1/FVC were consistent with an insignificant response to the bronchodilator (less than 12% improvement in FEV_1 and less than 200-mL increase in FEV_1 and/or FVC). To prepare for the educational session with this patient you must decide whether this patient's spirometric values represent obstructive or restrictive lung disease. What diagnostic test could further support your assessment?

2. You are reviewing the medical records of a 48-year-old male patient prior to performing a pulmonary function test. The patient's history and physical include current treatment for pulmonary sarcoidosis. The ordering physician has requested that this patient's pulmonary disease be verified as primarily obstructive or restrictive.
   A. Which pulmonary function tests will you choose to use to evaluate this patient?

B. What values will give you the most useful information?

KEY CONCEPT QUESTIONS

*Instructions: Choose the **single** best answer for each multiple choice question.*

1. Of the following, the **only** lung volume that can be measure by *direct* spirometry is:
   A. Residual volume (RV)
   B. Functional residual capacity (FRC)
   C. Vital capacity (VC)
   D. Total lung capacity (TLC)

2. The end-point of the helium dilution FRC test occurs when:
   A. Helium concentration in the lung is lowest
   B. Helium concentration in the spirometer is highest
   C. Helium is eliminated from the spirometer-patient system
   D. Helium concentration is equal throughout the spirometer-patient system

3. The nitrogen washout FRC test is based on the assumption that:
   A. Nitrogen concentration in the lung is normally about 80%
   B. 100% of the oxygen in the lung can be washed out by nitrogen
   C. Nitrogen washout quantifies trapped air volume
   D. Spirometer-lung nitrogen concentrations will equilibrate during the test

4. Body plethysmography is based on Boyle's law, which states that when gas volume and pressure changes occur, initial volume times initial pressure equals:
   A. Final volume times initial pressure
   B. Final volume times final pressure
   C. Initial volume divided by final pressure
   D. Final volume divided by final pressure

5. The three most common variables used to distinguish between obstructive and restrictive pulmonary function patterns are:
   A. FVC, FEV_1, and FEV_1/FVC
   B. FVC, $FEF_{25\%-75\%}$, and FEV_1
   C. FVC, PEF, and FEV_1
   D. FVC, FEV_1, and PIF

6. An example of a restrictive pulmonary disease is:
   A. Bronchial tumor
   B. Emphysema
   C. Asthma
   D. Congestive heart failure

6 | Pulmonary Blood Flow

After reading this chapter, you will be able to:

- Identify how the pulmonary and systemic circulations differ anatomically and functionally.
- Explain how blood flow, pressure, and vascular resistance in the pulmonary circulation can be assessed through pulmonary artery catheterization.
- Differentiate between causes of high pulmonary artery pressure through data obtained from the pulmonary artery catheter.
- Identify how right and left ventricular pumping function can be assessed through pulmonary artery catheterization.
- Calculate pulmonary vascular resistance.
- Differentiate between passive and active factors that affect pulmonary vascular resistance.
- Explain how the pulmonary vasculature can accommodate great increases in blood flow during exercise without significantly raising blood pressure.
- Identify why hypoxemia affects the right ventricle differently than the left ventricle.
- Identify how hypoxic pulmonary vasoconstriction can be both beneficial and harmful.
- Explain why the hypoxic pulmonary vasoconstriction response is diminished in certain pulmonary diseases.
- Explain why inhaled vasodilators can bring about beneficial physiologic changes not possible through systemic administration routes.
- Explain why gravity creates three distinct physiologic blood flow zones in the lung, and how they differ physiologically from one another.
- Describe how mechanical and physiologic changes can convert a blood flow zone in the lung to a different type of zone.
- Explain why the match between blood flow and ventilation in an upright individual is different in the lung base than in the lung apex.
- Identify what kinds of circulatory abnormalities cause pulmonary edema.

KEY TERMS AND DEFINITIONS

Define and give the abbreviation for each of the following terms:

1. Pulmonary capillary wedge pressure

2. Pulmonary artery pressure

3. Left atrial pressure

4. Left ventricular end-diastolic pressure

5. Central venous pressure

6. Right atrial pressure

7. Pulmonary vascular resistance

8. Pulmonary artery end-diastolic pressure

9. Mean arterial pressure

10. Nitric oxide

11. Hypoxic pulmonary vasoconstriction

12. Acute respiratory distress syndrome

13. Ventilator-induced lung injury

14. Ventilation/perfusion ratio

MATCHING

1. *Match the pulmonary artery catheter part on the left with its intended use(s) on the right. (Note: Some parts may have more than one use.)*

_____ 1. Balloon

_____ 2. Thermistor

_____ 3. Proximal lumen

_____ 4. Distal lumen

A. Used to access true mixed venous blood
B. Used to calculate cardiac output
C. Used to measure central venous pressure (CVP)
D. Used to measure pulmonary artery pressure (PAP)
E. Used to measure pulmonary capillary wedge pressure (PCWP)
F. Used to flow-direct catheter during insertion
G. Used to measure left atrial pressure (LAP)

2. *Match the following descriptors with the appropriate zones of blood flow.*

_____ 1. Intermittent blood flow through alveolar capillaries

_____ 2. Continuous blood flow that is proportional to the difference between arterial and venous pressure

_____ 3. Alveoli are ventilated but have no blood flow

A. Zone I
B. Zone II
C. Zone III

SHORT ANSWER/CRITICAL THINKING QUESTIONS

1. Examine the pressure waveforms in Figure 6-4 from the textbook.
   Why does the PA (pulmonary artery) waveform have a much higher diastolic pressure than the right ventricle (diastolic pressure = lowest point of the waveform)?

2. Explain why PCWP is used to estimate left atrial and left ventricular end-diastolic pressure.

3. Again, examine the Figure 6-4 from the textbook: as shown, the PA diastolic pressure (PADP) is only a couple of mm Hg higher than the PCWP, which is normal because the direction of blood flow is from pulmonary artery to the left ventricle.) What type of vascular change might cause the PADP to elevate to much higher than normal pressures while the PCWP stays essentially the same?

4. Which is most affected by a high pulmonary vascular resistance (PVR): the pulmonary artery pressure or the pulmonary capillary wedge pressure? Explain your answer.

5. Hypoxic pulmonary vasoconstriction (HPV) occurs in regions of the lung that have no ventilation, that is hypoxic lung regions. In what way is HPV a physiologically beneficial mechanism?

6. Why might chronic alveolar hypoxia lead to right ventricular strain and possibly failure?

7. Define pulmonary *shunt* and *dead space*. Explain the relationship of *shunt* and *dead space* to the ventilation/perfusion ratio ($\dot{V}/\dot{Q}$); that is high $\dot{V}/\dot{Q}$ and low $\dot{V}/\dot{Q}$ are associated with which conditions: shunt or dead space? Which portion of the upright lung tends to have the greatest amount of dead-space-like ventilation?

8. In what type of physiologic circumstances might breathing nitric oxide be beneficial? What is nitric oxide's effect on the cardiopulmonary system?

9. Refer to Figure 6-10 from the textbook.
   Explain why positive pressure mechanical ventilation may change Zone 3 pulmonary blood flow conditions to Zone 2 conditions, and Zone 2 conditions to Zone 1 conditions.

10. Which is most likely to cause an abnormally high PCWP: pumping failure of the left ventricle or high pulmonary artery pressure due to hypoxic pulmonary vasoconstriction? Which is most likely to cause *pulmonary edema* (fluid movement from pulmonary capillary blood to the interstitial spaces or into alveoli)? What *type* of pulmonary edema would this be? (See discussion of Pulmonary Edema in Clinical Focus 6-7 on page 127 in the textbook.)

CASE STUDIES

1. You have two patients that present with these cardiac pressure values:

   <u>Mr. K</u>
   PAP systolic = 38 mm Hg
   PAP diastolic = 25 mm Hg
   PCWP = 21 mm Hg

   <u>Mr. J</u>
   PAP systolic = 40 mm Hg
   PAP diastolic = 25 mm Hg
   PCWP = 10 mm Hg

   Mr. K and Mr. J have similarly high pulmonary artery pressures (35/25 and 40/25), but the causes of these high pressures are quite different.
   A. Compare and contrast the two different causes of high PAP, showing how the PCWP values help you come to your conclusions.

   B. Compare and contrast the different types of treatment that would be indicated in these two patients.

2. An ICU patient with a history of severe pulmonary emphysema has a pulmonary artery catheter in place. The patient's baseline hemodynamic pressures include a PCWP that is normal and PAP and CVP values that are above normal. The patient's chest x-ray reveals hyperinflation and right ventricular hypertrophy.
   A. Explain why the chest x-ray of a patient with severe pulmonary emphysema might show the presence of right ventricular enlargement (hypertrophy); drawing from your knowledge of the basic anatomic and physiologic defects of emphysema, explain the sequence of events that could lead to right ventricular hypertrophy.

B. Explain the etiology of the abnormal hemodynamic pressures in this patient.

C. What are some related physical examination abnormalities that might be produced by this situation?

KEY CONCEPT QUESTIONS

*Instructions: Choose the **single** best answer for each multiple choice question.*

1. High positive end-expiratory pressure and extended inspiratory time may cause an elevated PVR. This occurs because:
   A. Shunt is increased
   B. Zone I lung volume is increased
   C. Zone III lung volume is increased
   D. Alveolar capillaries have collapsed

2. In cardiogenic pulmonary edema, fluid accumulates in interstitial spaces primarily because of:
   A. Increased hydrostatic pressure
   B. Increased capillary permeability
   C. Decreased plasma oncotic pressure
   D. Increased fluid oncotic pressure

3. Causes for abnormally high PAP accompanying an abnormally high PCWP in a hypoxic patient include:
   A. Hypovolemia and pulmonary vasoconstriction
   B. Hypovolemia and mitral valve stenosis
   C. Left ventricular failure and pulmonary vasoconstriction
   D. Hypervolemia and low left ventricular preload

4. If a malpositioned pulmonary artery catheter resides in the pulmonary artery but cannot be adjusted to obtain a PCWP, the best estimation for this pressure (assuming PVR is normal) is:
   A. Systolic pulmonary artery pressure
   B. Central venous pressure
   C. Mean pulmonary artery pressure
   D. Diastolic pulmonary artery pressure

7 Gas Diffusion

OBJECTIVES

After reading this chapter, you will be able to:

- Differentiate between diffusion and bulk gas flow.
- Identify how to use the alveolar gas equation.
- Identify why the respiratory exchange ratio affects the calculation of alveolar oxygen pressure (PAO_2).
- Identify what factors affect diffusion, as illustrated by Fick's law.
- Identify how to use Graham's law and Henry's law to explain the differences in O_2 and CO_2 diffusion rates in the lung.
- Explain why O_2 transfer from lung to blood is perfusion limited, whereas CO transfer is diffusion limited.
- Identify why CO and not O_2 is the test gas normally used for measuring the lung's diffusion capacity.
- Explain how diffusion capacity is measured in a pulmonary function laboratory.
- Correlate disease entities with the abnormal processes that decrease diffusion rate.
- Explain why the diffusion capacity of the lung for carbon monoxide (D_LCO) test detects oxygenation problems in the natural progression of disease before abnormalities in arterial blood oxygen pressure (PaO_2) are evident.

KEY TERMS AND DEFINITIONS

Define the following abbreviations/terms:

1. Alveolar air equation

2. Diffusion

3. Fick's law

4. Graham's law

5. PAO_2

6. P_IO_2

7. Polycythemia

8. Respiratory exchange ratio (R)

9. Single-breath CO diffusion test (D_LCO_{SB})

10. Diffusion path length

11. Diffusion surface area

MATCHING

Match the value on the left with the appropriate normal sea-level partial pressure gradient on the right:

_____ 1. 0 mm Hg

_____ 2. 6 mm Hg

_____ 3. 40 mm Hg

_____ 4. 46 mm Hg

_____ 5. 47 mm Hg

_____ 6. 60 mm Hg

_____ 7. 100 mm Hg

_____ 8. 160 mm Hg

A. Carbon dioxide alveolar-capillary diffusion gradient
B. Oxygen partial pressure in inspired air
C. Alveolar carbon dioxide partial pressure
D. Capillary carbon dioxide partial pressure
E. Alveolar oxygen partial pressure
F. Oxygen alveolar-capillary diffusion gradient
G. Carbon dioxide partial pressure in inspired air
H. Alveolar water vapor partial pressure

LABELING

1. Using the illustration below, identify each of the following:

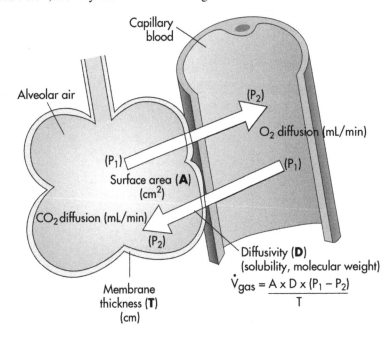

A. The gas that is represented by each arrow

B. The alveolar partial pressure of each gas at sea level

C. The normal volume of diffusion for each gas in mL/min

2. Using the illustrations below, answer each of the following questions:

Figure A

Oxygen Diffusion at Rest

$F_iO_2 = 0.21$

Mixed venous blood

$P_{\bar{v}}O_2 = 40$ mm Hg

$P_AO_2 = 100$ mm Hg

40

75

100

$PO_2 = 100$ mm Hg

Red blood cell:
75% saturated
with O_2

End-capillary blood

$PO_2 = 100$ mm Hg

Red blood cell:
98% saturated
with O_2

Enter
capillary

Leave
capillary

0   0   0.25   0.5   0.75

Capillary transit time (second)

Figure B

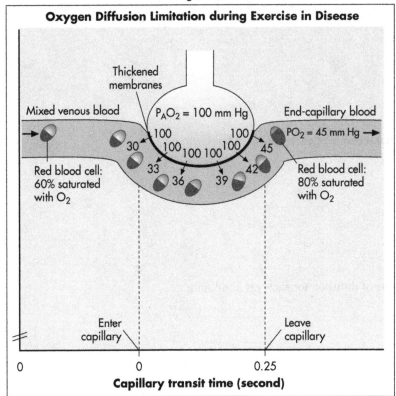

Oxygen Diffusion Limitation during Exercise in Disease

Thickened membranes

Mixed venous blood

$P_AO_2 = 100$ mm Hg

End-capillary blood

100   100
30   100 100 100 100   45 $PO_2 = 45$ mm Hg →

Red blood cell: 60% saturated with O_2

33
36   39   42

Red blood cell: 80% saturated with O_2

Enter capillary

Leave capillary

0   0   0.25

Capillary transit time (second)

A. Which figure depicts PO_2 equilibrium being reached between the alveolus and capillary?

B. What two effects would exercise have on the diffusion of oxygen in figure A (in a healthy lung)?

C. What is the explanation for the rapid rise to equilibrium in figure A?

D. Figure B depicts oxygen transport during exercise in a patient with lung disease. What has happened to the diffusion of oxygen across the alveolar-capillary membrane? Why?

E. Why does exercise highlight diffusion limitations in people who have certain types of lung disease (as depicted in figure B)?

3. Label each of the sites along the alveolar-capillary membrane diffusion pathway and identify which gas (O_2 or CO_2) is indicated by each of the arrows.

A. _____

B. _____

C. _____

D. _____

E. _____

F. _____

G. _____

H. _____

I. _____

J. _____

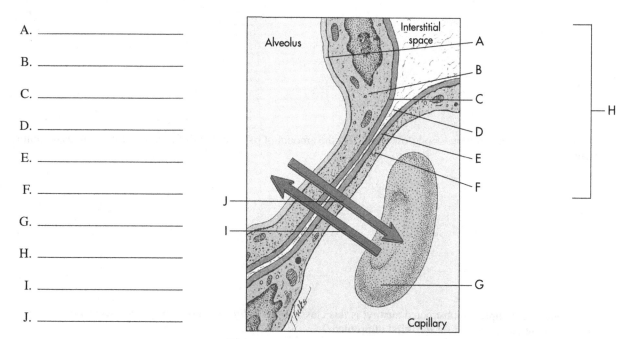

(From Seeley RR, Stephens TD, Tate P: *Anatomy & physiology,* ed 3, New York, 1995, McGraw-Hill.)

1. What does an R = 0.8 mean with respect to the volume of oxygen diffusing out of the lung compared to the volume of CO_2 entering the lung?

2. Calculate the PAO_2 of a person at sea level breathing 30% oxygen who has a CO_2 of 40 mm Hg (show your work).

3. Does oxygen or carbon dioxide diffuse more rapidly across the alveolar-capillary membrane? Why?

4. Does an increase in capillary blood flow rate affect the amount of oxygen that diffuses out of the lung each minute? Explain.

5. A person has a completely obstructed airway; is this classified as a *diffusion* problem? If not, what would be a more accurate classification for this kind of problem?

6. People with severe emphysema have low pulmonary diffusion capacity for oxygen even though diffusion path length may be normal at all points. Explain.

7. In normal, healthy people, oxygen diffusion from alveolar to capillary blood does not occur during most of the time blood is in contact with the alveolus. Why is this so?

8. Give an example of a condition in which oxygen diffusion rate would be purely *diffusion* limited and explain how that condition causes the diffusion defect.

9. *Chose the correct response from the two choices provided in the parentheses.*

   Our goal in measuring the lung's diffusion capacity is to find out how much the alveolar-capillary membrane resists diffusion of gas molecules from alveolar air to capillary blood. Therefore, we want pulmonary blood flow rate to (**affect/not affect**) the diffusion rate of our test gas. For this reason, we want the blood leaving the alveolar capillary to be (**fully saturated/far below saturation**) by the test gas. Why? Given the answers above, explain why carbon monoxide is the ideal gas for testing the diffusion capacity of the lung.

10. Although pulmonary interstitial edema increases diffusion path distance, this is probably **not** the mechanism by which pulmonary edema causes hypoxemia at rest. If this is the case, then what **is** the cause of hypoxemia due to pulmonary interstitial edema?

11. Explain why, during the course of progressive alveolar-capillary membrane thickening in lung disease, the D_LCO test will reveal abnormality before the measured PaO_2?

CASE STUDIES

1. As the respiratory therapist caring for an 88-year-old postoperative hip repair patient, you are consulted by a physical therapist regarding the patient's ability to ambulate. With a portable pulse oximeter, you note that the patient's oxygen saturation is significantly below normal on room air. The patient is still on 2 liters of oxygen by nasal cannula since surgery 4 days earlier and is only now starting to ambulate because of poor pain control. The patient's medical history is negative for any pulmonary or cardiac disease or treatment. The postoperative course includes inability to wean off of supplemental oxygen, immobility for approximately 96 hours, below normal inspiratory volumes measured during incentive spirometry, and bilateral inspiratory crackles upon auscultation. Without the benefit of D_LCO test results:

   A. What is your assumption about the patient's diffusion capacity?

   B. What is the cause of diffusion abnormalities in this patient?

C. What corrective actions can be taken?

2. You are a respiratory therapist working with a pulmonologist to perform routine annual health appraisals on-site at a large coal mining facility. A worker appears for her appointment with the chief complaint of "tiredness and lack of energy." You note that her spirometry results are consistent with restrictive lung disease and that her pulse oximetry demonstrates normal oxygen hemoglobin saturation at rest. Auscultation reveals bilateral fine inspiratory crackles. The patient tells you she recently completed a pulmonary stress test that indicated sub-optimal oxygenation during exercise. The pulmonologist asks you if you believe a follow-up appointment for a D_LCO test is indicated. What D_LCO test results would you expect to find with this patient and why?

KEY CONCEPT QUESTIONS

Instructions: *For the diffusion capacity defects below, label each as an example of increased diffusion path distance (P), decreased diffusion surface area (S), decreased uptake by red blood cells (U), or ventilation/perfusion mismatch (M).*

1. Anemia _____

2. Interstitial fibrosis _____

3. Engorged capillaries _____

4. High carbon monoxide blood levels _____

5. Destruction of alveolar-capillary bed _____

6. Regional atelectasis _____

7. Pulmonary embolus _____

8. Lobar pneumonia _____

*Instructions for multiple choice questions: Choose the **single** best answer for each multiple choice question.*

9. According to the alveolar air equation, all other factors remaining constant, PAO_2:
   A. Increases as $PACO_2$ increases
   B. Increases as P_IO_2 increases
   C. Decreases as the respiratory exchange ratio increases
   D. Decreases as inspired nitrogen decreases

10. Diffusion capacity increases toward normal after a hypervolemic patient with congestive left heart failure is given diuretic therapy. This improvement occurs because:
    A. The diffusion surface area is increased
    B. The low ventilation/perfusion ratio is corrected
    C. Red blood cell uptake is improved
    D. The diffusion path distance is decreased

11. Administering fluid to a severely dehydrated, hypotensive patient improves diffusion capacity because:
    A. Diffusion surface area is increased
    B. The low ventilation/perfusion ratio is corrected
    C. Red blood cell uptake is improved
    D. Diffusion path distance is decreased

12. We give patients with retained secretions humidified gas to breathe, improving their ability to cough out secretions and open previously plugged airways. Opening these airways improves diffusion capacity because:
    A. The diffusion surface area is increased
    B. The low ventilation/perfusion ratio is corrected
    C. The red blood cell uptake is improved
    D. The diffusion path distance is decreased

13. A D_LCO test result shows abnormally low diffusion for a patient with chronic hyperinflation, a significant smoking history, and dependence on supplemental oxygen. The clinical picture indicates the low diffusion rate is due to:
    A. The decreased diffusion surface area
    B. A low ventilation/perfusion ratio
    C. Decreased red blood cell uptake
    D. Increased diffusion path distance

Chapter **7** **Gas Diffusion**

8 Oxygen Equilibrium and Transport

OBJECTIVES

After reading this chapter, you will be able to:

- Describe how the blood takes up, transports, and releases oxygen.
- Explain the difference between arterial and venous oxygen contents and how they are related to oxygen consumption and cardiac output.
- Identify how oxygen content, oxygen saturation, oxygen partial pressure, and hemoglobin concentration are related to each other.
- Explain why the hemoglobin-oxygen binding process produces a sigmoid-shaped rather than linear PO_2-hemoglobin equilibrium curve.
- Explain why the sigmoid-shaped oxyhemoglobin equilibrium curve is physiologically advantageous.
- Describe how various factors affect the release and binding of oxygen by changing hemoglobin's affinity for oxygen.
- Explain why a change in the value of P_{50} means hemoglobin's affinity for oxygen has changed.
- Identify why cardiac output changes affect mixed venous PO_2, the difference between arterial and mixed venous oxygen content, and the amount of oxygen the tissues extract from the arterial blood each minute.
- Calculate the oxygen delivery rate, oxygen consumption, and tissue oxygen-extraction percentage.
- Explain why the PaO_2 and SaO_2 are insufficient indicators of tissue oxygenation.
- Explain why the PaO_2 is a more sensitive indicator than the SaO_2 of changes in the lung's ability to oxygenate the blood.
- Define critical oxygen delivery threshold.
- Explain why cyanosis may be absent in people who have high percentages of desaturated hemoglobin and why cyanosis may be present in people who have normal arterial oxygen contents.
- Describe how anemia caused by low hemoglobin content differs physiologically from anemia produced by carbon monoxide poisoning.
- Identify how fetal hemoglobin, methemoglobin, and sickle cell hemoglobin differ physiologically from normal hemoglobin.

KEY TERMS AND DEFINITIONS

Define the following terms:

1. Oxyhemoglobin

2. Deoxyhemoglobin

3. Arterial oxygen saturation (SaO_2)

4. Mixed venous oxygen saturation ($S_{\bar{v}}O_2$)

5. Anemia

6. Polycythemia

7. HbO_2 equilibrium curve

8. Arterial oxygen content (CaO_2)

9. Affinity

10. Bohr effect

11. Arterial-venous oxygen content difference ($C_{(a-\bar{v})}O_2$)

12. Oxygen-extraction ratio (O_2 ER)

13. Oxygen delivery (DO_2)

14. Oxygen consumption ($\dot{V}O_2$)

15. Critical oxygen delivery threshold (DO_2 crit)

16. Cyanosis

17. Carboxyhemoglobin

18. Fetal hemoglobin (HbF)

19. Methemoglobin (metHb)

20. Sickle cell hemoglobin (HbS)

MATCHING

Match the normal value on the right to the appropriate descriptor on the left.

_____ 1. Volume of O_2 for each gram of Hb

_____ 2. Total arterial oxygen content

_____ 3. Total venous oxygen content

_____ 4. Arterial-venous oxygen content difference

_____ 5. Oxygen extraction ratio

_____ 6. Dissolved arterial oxygen content

_____ 7. Dissolved venous oxygen content

A. 20 mL/dL
B. 5 mL/dL
C. 0.25
D. 0.3 mL/dL
E. 15 mL/dL
F. 1.34 mL
G. 0.12 mL/dL

LABELING

On the graph below, draw the oxyhemoglobin curves representing right and left shift and label each curve with the factors that cause its deviation from normal.

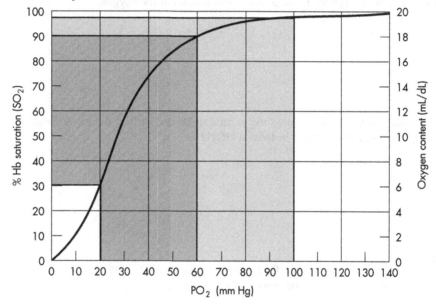

Refer to the figure above and circle the correct response:
1. A right shift of the oxyhemoglobin curve (***increases/decreases***) oxygen delivery to the tissue by (***increasing/decreasing***) plasma PO_2
2. A left shift of the oxyhemoglobin curve (***increases/decreases***) hemoglobin's affinity for oxygen and results in (***increased/decreased***) plasma PO_2

Chapter **8 Oxygen Equilibrium and Transport**

1. Explain how it is possible for arterial oxygen saturation percentage to be normal, and yet arterial oxygen content is low.

2. Why does giving 28% oxygen to a severely hypoxemic person (PaO_2 = 30 mm Hg) result in a larger increase in blood oxygen content than giving the same oxygen concentration to a person with a PaO_2 = 55 mm Hg?

3. Define P_{50} and explain how it is related to the affinity of hemoglobin for oxygen.

4. In the body at the tissue level, what effect does the normal rightward shift of the oxyhemoglobin equilibrium curve have on plasma PO_2? In what way is this a beneficial effect?

5. Calculate oxygen delivery rate in mL/min:
   Hb = 9 g/dL   Cardiac output = 5.5 L/min PaO_2 = 95 mm Hg SaO_2 = 97%
   Is this a normal O_2 delivery rate? What is the nature of the problem?

6. See #5 above: If mixed venous PO_2 = 43 mm Hg and $S_{\bar{v}}O_2$ = 76%.
   A. What is the tissue oxygen extraction (consumption) in L/min?

B. What percentage is this of oxygen delivery?

C. What is the normal tissue O_2 extraction percentage (also known as the O_2 extraction ratio)?

7. Explain the way in which cardiac output affects mixed venous oxygen content and the arterial-venous oxygen content difference.

CASE STUDIES

1. You are called to the ER to draw a blood gas from a patient who sustained multiple injuries in a motor vehicle accident. The results of the blood gas are as follows:

PaO_2 = 75 mm Hg

$PaCO_2$ = 58 mm Hg

pH = 7.28

SaO_2 = 88%

Temp = 37° C

A. Normally, what oxygen saturation is associated with a PaO_2 of 75 mm Hg?

B. With regard to the oxyhemoglobin dissociation curve, what conclusions can be drawn from this blood gas?

2. A postoperative cardiac patient has just arrived to the coronary care unit. After 30 minutes of mechanical ventilation, you draw a blood gas and perform cardiac output measurements. The results are as follows:

PaO_2 = 65 mm Hg
$PaCO_2$ = 40 mm Hg
pH = 7.40
Hb = 13 g/dL
SaO_2 = 98%
CO = 4.8 L/min
Is this patient adequately oxygenated? Explain.

KEY CONCEPT QUESTIONS

*Instructions: Choose the **single** best answer for each multiple choice question.*

1. Between 10 and 40 mm Hg PO_2 on the oxyhemoglobin curve:
   A. Oxygen content changes little for each unit of change in PO_2
   B. Oxygen is normally unloading from hemoglobin
   C. A safety margin exists for oxygen content as PaO_2 decreases
   D. Oxygen is normally loading on hemoglobin

2. A high P_{50} means that:
   A. More than 50 mm Hg is required to saturate 50% of hemoglobin
   B. Less than 50 mm Hg is required to saturate 50% of hemoglobin
   C. More oxygen is loaded on hemoglobin than at a normal P_{50}
   D. Hemoglobin affinity for oxygen is advantageous for tissue oxygenation

3. A patient with a hemoglobin concentration of 8.0 has an SaO_2 of 94%. Which of the following improves the patient's oxygen delivery more:
   A. Increasing the SaO_2 to 100% by adding supplemental oxygen
   B. Increasing the hemoglobin concentration to 10 g/dL by transfusing blood

4. An adequately hydrated patient has a hemoglobin concentration of 15, an SaO_2 of 97%, a PaO_2 of 98 mm Hg, a cardiac output of 2.8 L/min, and a venous oxygen content of 9.5 mL/dL. The low venous oxygen content is the result of:
   A. Low hemoglobin
   B. Low arterial oxygen content
   C. Hypovolemia
   D. Low cardiac output

9 Carbon Dioxide Equilibrium and Transport

OBJECTIVES

After reading this chapter, you will be able to:

- Explain how blood levels of PCO_2, dissolved CO_2, carbonic acid, and alveolar ventilation are interrelated.
- Identify how blood levels of CO_2 play a role in the body's acid-base balance.
- Use the CO_2 hydration reaction to explain how changes in alveolar ventilation affect blood levels of CO_2 and hydrogen ions.
- Identify why equal CO_2 production and elimination rates can coexist with normal ventilation, hypoventilation, or hyperventilation.
- Explain how CO_2 is transported in different ways in the blood plasma and erythrocytes.
- Identify how hemoglobin in the erythrocyte helps generate plasma bicarbonate ions (HCO_3^-).
- Explain how the Bohr and Haldane effects are mutually enhancing with regard to oxygen and carbon dioxide transport.

KEY TERMS AND DEFINITIONS

Define the following terms:

1. Carbonic acid (H_2CO_3)

2. Carbonic anhydrase

3. Chemical equilibrium

4. Chloride shift

5. CO_2 hydration reaction

6. Haldane effect

7. Law of mass action

MATCHING

Match the following values with the appropriate statement. Values may be used more than once.

_____ 1. Normal tissue PCO_2

_____ 2. Normal alveolar PCO_2 (P_ACO_2)

_____ 3. Normal blood $PaCO_2$

_____ 4. Normal dissolved PCO_2 in arterial blood

A. 40 mm Hg
B. 46 mm Hg
C. 1.2 mmol/L

73

*Indicate whether each of the following statements occurs during **hyperventilation(hyper)** or **hypoventilation(hypo)**.*

_____ 1. Alveolar PCO_2 increases

_____ 2. H_2CO_3 increases

_____ 3. Dissolved CO_2 increases

_____ 4. Plasma PCO_2 increases

_____ 5. Plasma PCO_2 decreases

_____ 6. Right-shifted hydration reaction

_____ 7. Left-shifted hydration reaction

LABELING
Label the figure below by filling in the appropriate normal resting values for CO_2 production, CO_2 elimination, alveolar CO_2, and plasma CO_2.

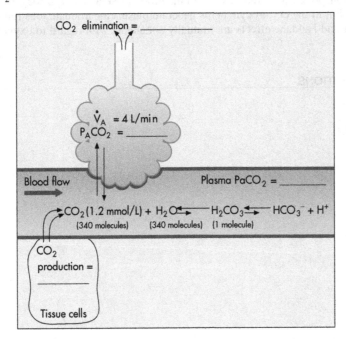

SHORT ANSWER/CRITICAL THINKING QUESTIONS

1. Write the chemical reaction showing how CO_2 in the blood plasma generates hydrogen ions (H^+).

2. Explain why alveolar ventilation affects the hydrogen ion concentration (H^+) in the blood.

3. Refer to the reaction in #1 above: compare the speed of this reaction in blood plasma with its speed inside the erythrocyte, and explain why the speeds are different.

4. When CO_2 diffuses out of the body's tissue cells into the capillary blood, most of it (95%) immediately enters the erythrocyte, as though it is somehow actively drawn in. What events inside the erythrocyte cause CO_2 to diffuse into the erythrocyte so readily, leaving only 5% behind in the plasma?

5. When CO_2 diffuses into the erythrocyte, bicarbonate ions (HCO_3^-) build up inside the erythrocyte and eventually diffuse out into the plasma. What mechanisms are responsible for this event?

6. In what way does CO_2's attachment to the hemoglobin molecule affect hemoglobin's affinity for O_2? What is the name of this "effect"? Explain how this effect enhances the gas exchange occurring at the tissue level.

Chapter **9** **Carbon Dioxide Equilibrium and Transport**

7. List all forms in which CO_2 is carried in the blood, listing them in order from most prevalent to least prevalent.

8. Compare the CO_2 blood equilibrium curve with that of O_2. What is the most striking difference in the shapes of the curves? Use these curves to explain why alveolar ventilation affects blood content of CO_2 differently than it affects blood O_2 content.

9. In what way does hemoglobin's saturation with oxygen affect the blood's capacity to carry carbon dioxide? What is the name for this "effect"? Explain how this effect enhances the gas exchange that occurs at the alveolar level.

CASE STUDY

1. A cardiac arrest patient who was successfully resuscitated has just been placed on mechanical ventilation. The ICU physician orders an arterial blood gas (ABG) to be drawn 30 minutes after initiation of mechanical ventilation. Thirty minutes later, the ABG reveals a PO_2 of 110 mm Hg, a PCO_2 of 38 mm Hg, and a pH of 7.25. A laboratory blood sample reveals very high lactic acid levels following the resuscitative efforts. The attending physician requests your input to appropriately change the patient's ventilator parameters.

   A. What would you suggest?

B. How can changing the patient's ventilation improve this patient's clinical picture?

2. Two hours after you made ventilator changes, including an increase in the number of breaths per minute delivered by the ventilator, a follow-up ABG reveals a PO_2 of 115 mm Hg, a PCO_2 of 29 mm Hg, and a pH of 7.5. Since the physician left instructions to "titrate breathing frequency according to blood gas results," is there a change indicated and, if so, what change(s) would you make?

KEY CONCEPT QUESTIONS

*Instructions: Choose the **single** best answer for each multiple choice question.*

1. Carbon dioxide is produced:
   A. As a by-product of aerobic metabolic activity of body tissues
   B. As a by-product of anaerobic metabolic activity of body tissues
   C. As a consequence of carbonic acid formation in body tissues
   D. As a consequence of elevated H^+ ion concentrations in body tissues

2. If tissue metabolism increases and alveolar ventilation remains normal, which of the following will occur?
   A. $PaCO_2$ will increase
   B. Ph will increase
   C. H_2CO_3 will decrease
   D. H^+ ion concentration will decrease

3. Which of the following is consistent with an acidic state secondary to decreased ventilation?
   A. $P_ACO_2 < 40$ mm Hg
   B. $PaCO_2 < 40$ mm Hg
   C. Increased blood carbonic acid
   D. Low H^+ ion concentration

4. An arterial blood gas analysis of a patient breathing room air provides these results: $PaO_2 = 55$ mm Hg and $PaCO_2 = 34$ mm Hg. Without other clinical data, this information suggests that the patient:
   A. Is hypoxemic secondary to hypoventilation
   B. Has chronic obstructive airways disease with alveolar CO_2 retention
   C. Is hyperventilating secondary to hypoxemia
   D. Has a blood carbonic acid level above normal

10 Acid-Base Regulation

OBJECTIVES

After reading this chapter, you will be able to:

- Explain how hydrogen ion concentration [H^+] affects cellular enzyme activity.
- Define acid and base according to the Brønsted-Lowry classification scheme.
- Explain how the strength of an acid and its equilibrium or ionization constant are related.
- Explain the relationship between the concept of pH and H^+ ion concentration.
- Explain how isohydric buffering in the blood prevents large pH changes when CO_2 reacts with water to form carbonic acid.
- Identify why bicarbonate and nonbicarbonate buffer systems differ in their ability to buffer volatile and fixed acids.
- Derive the Henderson-Hasselbalch equation from the ionization constant for carbonic acid.
- Explain why the body's open and closed buffer systems differ in their ability to buffer fixed and volatile acids.
- Use the Henderson-Hasselbalch equation to predict the change in ventilation required to produce a given arterial pH.
- Use the Henderson-Hasselbalch equation to calculate the pH, [HCO_3^-], and PCO_2.
- Use arterial blood-gas values to distinguish between primary respiratory and primary metabolic acid-base disturbances.
- Identify what the body's compensatory responses are to primary respiratory and metabolic acid-base disturbances.
- Explain why acute changes in PCO_2 affect blood levels of HCO_3^-.

KEY TERMS AND DEFINITIONS

Define the following terms:

1. Cations

2. Anions

3. Buffers

4. Acidosis

5. Alkalosis

6. Fixed acid

7. Conjugate base

8. Buffer solution

9. Buffer base

10. Open buffer system

11. Closed buffer system

12. Isohydric principle

13. Dissociation

MATCHING

Match the symbols on the right to the correct term on the left.

_____ 1. Hydrogen ion concentration

_____ 2. Base component

_____ 3. Carbonic acid

_____ 4. Bicarbonate

_____ 5. Hydrochloric acid

_____ 6. Sodium hydroxide

_____ 7. Sodium bicarbonate

A. H_2CO_3
B. H^+
C. HCO_3^-
D. HCl
E. NaOH
F. $NaHCO_3$
G. OH^-

SHORT ANSWER/CRITICAL THINKING QUESTIONS

1. Define the terms *acid* and *base* according to the Brønsted-Lowry theory.

2. Explain the concepts of *fixed* versus *volatile* acids in the body.

3. Explain what is meant by the term *equilibrium constant* with regard to an acid, and describe *strong* and *weak* acids in terms of their equilibrium constants.

4. Finish the equation expressing pH in terms of hydrogen ion (H^+) concentration:

   pH = _____

5. The normal *range* for arterial blood pH is _____ which corresponds to an H^+ concentration range of _____. A fall in pH of one unit corresponds to an H^+ concentration *(increase/decrease?)* by a factor of _____.

6. A *buffer* consists of an acid and its _____ as illustrated in the reaction (bold items are the two components of the buffer): $\mathbf{H_2CO_3} \leftrightharpoons H^+ + \mathbf{HCO_3^-}$

7. Show how the reaction between CO_2 and H_2O in the blood plasma functions as a buffer when H^+ of a fixed are added to the plasma:
   $$CO_2 + H_2O \leftrightharpoons H_2CO_3 \leftrightharpoons HCO_3^- + H^+$$
   What is the name of this buffer system? _____ Is this an example of an open or a closed buffer system?

8. What is the advantage of an open buffer system over a closed system in buffering fixed acids?

9. Write the Henderson-Hasselbalch equation, and solve it for arterial blood pH using normal values for $PaCO_2$ (40 mm Hg) and $[HCO_3^-]$ (24 mEq/L). What is the ratio between dissolved CO_2 and HCO_3^- concentration in this instance?

10. When a buffer is dissociated such that it consists of 50% acid molecules and 50% base molecules, the system's pH

    is referred to as the system's _____. Under such conditions, the buffer's ability to resist pH changes when acids or bases are added to it is (*greatest/least?*).

11. List the main *non-bicarbonate* buffers in the blood. Which is the most important non-bicarbonate buffer? Are these buffers considered *open* or *closed* systems?

12. Respiratory acidosis occurs when the lungs _____ which causes the

    _____ in the arterial blood to rise. Write the chemical reaction illustrating this situation: As long as the lungs continue to function abnormally in this manner, the reaction above will continue to move to the (*right/left?*) and respiratory acidosis will persist. In this case, only one type of buffer system is able to buffer the acid produced, which is the (*bicarbonate/non-bicarbonate?*) system.

13. The two organ systems that regulate acid-base balance of the blood are the _____ and

    the _____. *Respiratory* acidosis or alkalosis can be countered or *compensated* by the

    actions of the _____ while *non-respiratory* acidosis or alkalosis can be compensated

    by the actions of the _____. In both cases, compensatory actions work to maintain a

    normal blood _____.

14. Compensated respiratory acidosis would be characterized by a high _____ (the primary

    problem) and a high _____ (the compensatory response). Compensated metabolic

    (non-respiratory) acidosis would be characterized by a low _____ (the primary

    problem) and a low _____ (the compensatory response).

15. *Fill in the Blanks:*

Primary Problem	Compensatory Response	Classification of the Abnormality
High HCO_3^-	_____	compensated metabolic alkalosis
High $PaCO_2$	Renal HCO_3^- retention	_____
_____	Hypoventilation	compensated metabolic acidosis
_____	Renal HCO_3^- excretion	_____

16. The plasma HCO_3^- concentration rises slightly when $PaCO_2$ rises acutely "this is explained by events occurring in the erythrocyte. As CO_2 diffuses in, the H^+ generated by the CO_2 hydration reaction is immediately buffered by

_____" which generates HCO_3^- inside the erythrocyte, which eventually diffuses into the

plasma. For every acute 10 mm Hg rise in $PaCO_2$, the plasma HCO_3^- rises by about _____ mEq/L.

CASE STUDIES

1. A 74-year-old male is in the intensive care unit after suffering a stroke and has been placed on mechanical ventilation. Arterial blood gas measurements from the patient reveal the following:

pH	7.50
$PaCO_2$	40 mm Hg
PaO_2	95 mm Hg
SaO_2	98%
HCO_3^-	24 mEq/L

A. How would you interpret this patient's acid-base status?

B. What do you think is causing this acid-base abnormality?

C. How does this patient's hyperventilation pattern raise the pH of the blood?

D. How might the kidneys respond to this acid-base disturbance?

2. A 30-year-old female has been having symptoms of the flu for the past week. She has been vomiting several times every day and is having a difficult time keeping solids and liquids down; the result is severe dehydration. After a fainting episode at work, she was taken to a walk-in clinic, where an IV was placed to help rehydrate her. An arterial blood gas was drawn, revealing the following:

pH	7.50
$PaCO_2$	40 mm Hg
PaO_2	95 mm Hg
SaO_2	97%
HCO_3^-	32 mEq/L

A. How would you interpret her acid-base disturbance?

B. Why might excessive vomiting cause her particular acid-base disturbance?

C. Could the lungs compensate for this acid-base disturbance?

KEY CONCEPT QUESTIONS

*Instructions: Choose the **single** best answer for each multiple choice question.*

1. Alkalosis refers to:
   A. An accumulation of H^+ in body fluids
   B. Body fluids with subnormal pH
   C. Higher than normal amounts of proton acceptors in body fluids
   D. Reduced concentrations of base in body fluids

2. The lungs eliminate CO_2 produced by:
   A. The open buffer system only
   B. Fixed acids only
   C. Volatile and fixed acids
   D. Volatile acids only

3. When $PaCO_2$ is high, the kidneys excrete:
   A. Greater amounts of H^+ and smaller amounts of HCO_3^-
   B. Smaller amounts of H^+ and greater amounts of HCO_3^-
   C. Greater amounts of both H^+ and HCO_3^-
   D. Smaller amounts of both H^+ and HCO_3^-

4. Respiratory alkalosis is caused by:
   A. Decreased HCO_3^- excretion
   B. Increased CO_2 excretion
   C. Hypoventilation
   D. Increased dissolved CO_2

5. Metabolic acid-base disturbances are caused primarily by:
   A. Gains or losses in plasma HCO_3^- only
   B. Increases or decreases in dissolved CO_2
   C. Gains or losses of fixed acids or HCO_3^-
   D. Changes in the denominator of the Henderson-Hasselbalch equation

11 Control of Ventilation

OBJECTIVES

After reading this chapter, you will be able to:

- Explain how the medullary respiratory center generates the basic breathing pattern.
- Describe how the medullary respiratory neurons and pontine centers interact.
- Explain how various reflexes and receptors affect ventilation, including the Hering-Breuer inflation reflex, J-receptors, proprioceptors, and muscle spindles.
- Identify how CO_2 indirectly stimulates the medullary chemoreceptors.
- Explain why high arterial PCO_2 more readily stimulates the central chemoreceptors than high arterial levels of metabolically produced fixed acid.
- Identify why arterial PCO_2 is a more appropriate controller of ventilation than arterial PO_2.
- Explain why hypoxemia plays a more important role in regulating ventilation in patients with chronically high $PaCO_2$ than in patients with normal $PaCO_2$.
- Differentiate between the immediate and chronic effects of high altitude on ventilation and explain why they occur.
- Identify two mechanisms whereby oxygen administration might induce hypercapnia in patients who have severe chronic obstructive pulmonary disease.
- Explain how $PaCO_2$ affects the cerebral circulation and intracranial pressure.

KEY TERMS AND DEFINITIONS

Define the following terms:

1. Medulla oblongata

2. Pons

3. Apneustic center

4. Pneumotaxic center

5. Hering-Breuer reflex

6. Head's reflex

7. Chemoreceptors

8. Central chemoreceptors

9. Peripheral chemoreceptors

10. Apneustic breathing

11. Biot's breathing

12. Cheyne-Stokes breathing

MATCHING/FILL-IN-THE-BLANK

1. Match the respiratory center components on the left with their appropriate description. (Note: One description is used twice.)

_____ Apneustic center

_____ Dorsal respiratory group

_____ Ventral respiratory group

_____ Pneumotaxic center

A. Provide the main stimulus for inspiration
B. Has neural connections with the pneumotaxic center but is poorly understood
C. Found bilaterally in the medulla. Contains both inspiratory and expiratory neurons
D. Limits inspiration and holds apneustic signals in check

2. Match the terms on the left with their appropriate description.

_____ Hering-Breuer reflex

_____ J-receptors

_____ Vagovagal reflexes

_____ Deflation reflex

_____ Slowly adapting receptors

_____ Rapidly adapting irritant receptors

_____ Peripheral proprioceptors

A. Causes rapid shallow breathing and a sensation of dyspnea, when stimulated by inflammation, pulmonary vascular congestion, or edema
B. Located in muscles, tendons, and joints. Stimulated by exercise and pain
C. Stretch receptors that generate the Hering-Breuer reflex
D. Located in large airway epithelium. Stimulation causes cough, bronchospasm sneezing, and tachypnea
E. Responsible for rapid respiratory rate associated with sudden lung collapse
F. Reflexes with both sensory and motor vagal components
G. Only activated at large lung volumes in adults

3. Indicate whether each of the statements below is true regarding the central chemoreceptors (*central*) or peripheral chemoreceptors (*peripheral*) or *both*.

_____ Respond to arterial carbon dioxide, hypoxia, and hydrogen ions

_____ Are in direct contact with cerebral spinal fluid

_____ Located in the arch of the aorta and bifurcations of the carotid arteries

_____ Respond directly to changes in hydrogen ion concentration

_____ Respond to decreased arterial partial pressure of oxygen

_____ Account for 20% to 30% of the ventilatory response to hypercapnia

_____ Respond indirectly to changes in PCO_2

_____ Hypoxia increases sensitivity to hydrogen ion concentration

88

LABELING

Label the diagram of the brain stem with the names of its three main parts and the names of respiratory neuron groups; pneumotaxic center, apneustic center, medulla oblongata, pons, spinal cord, ventral respiratory groups, dorsal respiratory groups, nucleus ambiguus, and nucleus retroambiguus.

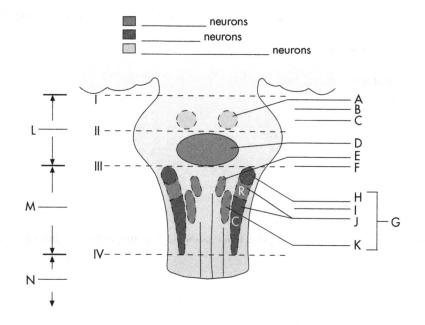

A. _____   F. _____   K. _____

B. _____   G. _____   L. _____

C. _____   H. _____   M. _____

D. _____   I. _____   N. _____

E. _____   J. _____

1. The rhythmic spontaneous breathing pattern is caused by nerve impulses originating in which part of the

   brain? _____ The nerve group containing *mainly inspiratory* neurons is known as the

   _____ _____ while the nerve group containing *both inspiratory*

   and expiratory neurons is known as the _____.

2. Which neurons are most active during basic, rhythmic breathing? Explain.

3. What is it about the inspiratory neuronal impulse that causes gradual lung expansion instead of an abrupt
   inspiratory gasp?

4. Which brain center controls the "off switch" point of the inspiratory ramp signal? Where in the brain is it located?
   How does this center accomplish "switching off" the inspiratory signal? What is the consequence of a weak
   signal from this center?

5. Which center, if unrestrained, generates strong signals resulting in prolonged inspiratory gasps?

6. Which reflex has an effect similar to that of the pneumotaxic center? Where are the receptors for this reflex located? Under what circumstances is this reflex most likely to play an important role in controlling the ventilatory pattern?

7. What are the body's responses to activation of the following reflexes:

   A. Vagovagal reflex

   B. J-receptor reflex

   Where are the receptors for these reflexes located?

8. Where are the central chemoreceptors located? To which chemical (specifically) are they sensitive? Why does elevated arterial blood carbon dioxide elicit a chemoreceptor response more quickly than elevated arterial hydrogen ion concentration?

9. Which chemoreceptors are responsive to hypoxemia? Where are they located? To which other chemicals do they respond?

10. Explain the way in which breathing high oxygen concentrations causes a chronically hypercapnic, hypoxemic patient to hypoventilate?

11. Why may it be beneficial to mechanically hyperventilate the head injury patient suffering from high intracranial pressure? Why is a hyperventilation strategy controversial in this instance? Why does this benefit diminish after 24 to 48 hours?

CASE STUDIES

1. A patient with chronic obstructive pulmonary disease (COPD) with chronic hypercapnia is on the orthopedic surgical unit after total hip replacement surgery. As the respiratory therapist responsible for this unit, you are providing the patient's maintenance regimen of inhaled bronchodilators and steroids. Because of the patient's pulmonary history, a preoperative arterial blood gas sample was drawn and analyzed while the patient was receiving oxygen by nasal cannula running at 1 L/min. Blood gas results at that time were: $PO_2 = 58$ mm Hg, $PCO_2 = 50$ mm Hg, $SaO_2 = 89\%$, pH = 7.36, and $HCO_3^- = 27.3$ mEq/L. Postoperatively the patient is receiving self-administered analgesics (pain relievers) for pain and is on supplemental oxygen at 1 L/min. On the first postoperative day, the patient's surgeon analyzes the electrolytes and notices that the total CO_2 (dissolved CO_2 and CO_2 carried as HCO_3^-) is above normal. The patient is alert and breathing at his normal rate of 20 breaths per minute. The surgeon requests that a blood gas be drawn to evaluate the patient's ventilatory status. The arterial blood gas results on 1 L/min oxygen are: $PO_2 = 59$ mm Hg, $PCO_2 = 51$ mm Hg, $SaO_2 = 89\%$, pH = 7.35, and $HCO_3^- = 27$ mEq/L. The surgeon reviews the blood gas results and, because the $PaCO_2$ is above normal, is concerned that the patient may be using excessive amounts of pain medication, thus depressing his drive to breathe. What is your assessment of the patient's ventilatory status?

2. The patient in the case above is now in his fourth postoperative day and is using only small amounts of pain medication. Physical therapists have been walking with the patient since the second postoperative day. One of the physical therapists pages you and asks you to evaluate the patient because of concerns about a change in the patient's condition. When you enter the room, you notice that the patient is lethargic and arouses only briefly when his name is spoken loudly. You also observe that the patient's nasal cannula is in place and that the oxygen liter flow has been increased to 3 L/min. A portable pulse oximeter probe attached to the patient's finger reveals an SpO_2 of 95% with a breathing frequency of 10. You reduce the oxygen flow to 1 L/min, continue to monitor the patient's ventilatory status, and page the physical therapist to let them know that the patient's condition should be improved enough to allow for exercise within the hour, pending a follow-up SpO_2 check. Explain your actions and your statement to the physical therapist.

KEY CONCEPT QUESTIONS

*Instructions: Choose the **single** best answer for each multiple choice question.*

1. A spinal cord injury that results in transection of the brain stem between the pons and medulla will result in which of the following?
   A. Cheyne-Stokes breathing
   B. Biot's breathing
   C. Irregular, spontaneous breathing
   D. Apnea

2. Central and peripheral chemoreceptors stimulate ventilation due to which of the following?
   A. Hypercapnia
   B. Hypoxia
   C. Alkalemia
   D. Both A and B

3. Hypoventilation accompanying closed head injuries and central nervous system damage may result in further brain damage because:
   A. Decreased $PaCO_2$ constricts cerebral vessels.
   B. Increased $PaCO_2$ lowers intracranial pressure.
   C. Increased blood $[H^+]$ dilates cerebral blood vessels.
   D. Decreased blood $[H^+]$ increases intracranial pressure

4. Painful stimuli and limb movement produce ventilation in patients with respiratory depression because of stimulatory signals sent by:
   A. Peripheral proprioreceptors
   B. Irritant receptors
   C. Rapidly adapting receptors
   D. Central chemoreceptors

12 Ventilation-Perfusion Relationships

After reading this chapter, you will be able to:

- Explain why alveolar ventilation ($\dot{V}_A$) and pulmonary capillary blood flow ($\dot{Q}_C$) determine the alveolar PO_2.
- Use the oxygen–carbon dioxide diagram to characterize absolute shunt and absolute dead space.
- Explain why there is an alveolar-arterial PO_2 difference in the normal lung.
- Identify why the $P(A\text{-}a)O_2$ increases as the fraction of inspired oxygen (F_IO_2) increases.
- Explain why high $\dot{V}_A/\dot{Q}_C$ lung regions can compensate for the hypercapnia but not the hypoxemia of low $\dot{V}_A/\dot{Q}_C$ regions.
- Differentiate between general hypoventilation, shunt, and $\dot{V}_A/\dot{Q}_C$ mismatch as causes of hypoxemia.
- Explain why absolute shunt is not responsive to oxygen therapy.
- Describe the major pathological defects involved in shunt and dead-space–producing diseases.
- Differentiate between the effects absolute shunt and absolute dead space have on arterial blood gases.
- Identify which of the following shunt indicators is the most clinically accurate and reliable: $P(A\text{-}a)O_2$, PaO_2/F_IO_2, or PaO_2/P_AO_2.
- Use the classic physiologic shunt equation to calculate the fraction of shunted cardiac output.
- Explain why changes in cardiac output affect PaO_2 in a patient with abnormally high intrapulmonary shunt.

KEY TERMS AND DEFINITIONS

Define the following terms:

1. $\dot{V}_A/\dot{Q}_c$ ratio

2. V/Q mismatching

3. Absolute shunt

4. Absolute dead space

5. Relative dead space

6. Relative shunt

7. Venous admixture

8. A-a gradient

9. a-A ratio

10. Oxygen ratio

MATCHING/FILL-IN-THE-BLANK

Match the term on the left to the correct description on the right.

_____ 1. Hypoventilation

_____ 2. V/Q mismatch

_____ 3. Shunt

A. Most common cause of hypoxemia
B. Hypoxemia not related to an oxygen-transfer problem
C. Abnormal process that prevents alveolar ventilation

4. For each of the following right-to-left shunting mechanisms, indicate whether it is an example of an anatomic (A) or intrapulmonary (P) shunt.

_____ Atelectasis

_____ Pulmonary edema

_____ Pneumonia

_____ Ventricular septal defect

_____ Bronchial occlusion

_____ Adult respiratory distress syndrome (ARDS)

_____ Airway mucus plug

_____ Pneumothorax

_____ Bronchial venous admixture

SHORT ANSWER/CRITICAL THINKING QUESTIONS

1. A young, previously healthy drug overdose victim in the emergency department presents with the following arterial blood gases (ABGs) while breathing room air:

    pH = 7.22
    PO_2 = 59 mm Hg
    PCO_2 = 63 mm Hg
    Barometric pressure = 760 mm Hg

    A. What is the mechanism causing this person's hypoxemia: *overall hypoventilation, V/Q mismatch,* or *absolute shunt?*

B. Calculate $P_{A}O_{2}$

C. Is there an oxygen transfer (alveolar gas to capillary blood) problem?

2. A patient diagnosed with COPD presents with these ABGs on room air (P_{B} = 730 mm Hg):
   pH = 7.45
   PO_{2} = 60 mm Hg
   PCO_{2} = 33 mm Hg
   A. What is the mechanism causing this person's hypoxemia: *overall hypoventilation, V/Q mismatch,* or *absolute shunt?* Can any of these mechanisms be immediately ruled out?

   B. This patient was given oxygen via nasal cannula at 2 L/min. The resulting PaO_{2} was 90 mm Hg. What is the predominant hypoxemic mechanism?

3. Examine Figure 12-8 in text.
   A. Why does breathing 100% oxygen fail to maximally saturate the arterial blood or significantly raise the arterial PO_{2} during absolute shunt?

B. Since raising the F_IO_2 is ineffective, what measures must be taken to improve the PaO_2 in this instance?

4. Examine Figure 12-9 in text. Note in both A and B of this figure, one alveolus has a $PCO_2 = 60$ mm Hg and the other a $PCO_2 = 20$ mm Hg and the *arterial* PCO_2 (which is a mixture of the blood from the two alveoli) is in the normal range (43 mm Hg). This means *hyperventilation* of "good" areas in the lung can compensate for high PCO_2s of poorly ventilated areas and produce normal-range arterial PCO_2s. But look at the alveolar PO_2s in **A** of this figure. The high PO_2 of the hyperventilated alveolus (125 mm Hg) cannot compensate for the low PO_2 (50 mm Hg) of the underventilated alveolus; that is, the arterial PO_2 (a mixture from both alveoli) is only 60 mm Hg, which is not the average of the two alveolar PO_2s. *This shows it is possible for arterial PCO_2 to be normal in the presence of arterial hypoxemia.* **Why can increased ventilation of normal alveoli compensate for high PCO_2s of poorly ventilated alveoli, but not for low PO_2s of poorly ventilated alveoli?**

5. Explain why alveolar dead space (alveoli that have lost their blood flow) produces the following:
   A. Very high minute ventilation, but a near normal $PaCO_2$

   B. An arterial-alveolar PCO_2 difference (i.e. $PaCO_2$ is greater than the average alveolar PCO_2)

6. Compare the three shunt indicators ($P(A-a)O_2$, PaO_2/P_AO_2, and PaO_2/F_IO_2) by answering the following questions:

A. Which is the most stable?

B. Which is actually an expression of the percentage of alveolar oxygen transferred into capillary blood?

C. Which is an unreliable estimator of shunt in the presence of hypoventilation (high PCO_2)?

7. Explain why a sudden decrease in cardiac output causes all three shunt indicators, ($P(A-a)O_2$, PaO_2/P_AO_2, and PaO_2/F_IO_2), to erroneously overestimate shunt percentage? In what way does a low cardiac output in the presence of shunt decrease arterial blood PO_2?

8. An ARDS patient has these blood gases and other values:

	Arterial	Venous	
PO_2	100	30	Hb = 15 g/dL
PCO_2	35	45	F_IO_2 = .8
Sat.%	98.5	60	P_B = 747 mm Hg

Calculate the physiologic shunt (see example in Clinical Focus 12-7 in the textbook).
In this example, what percentage of the cardiac output perfuses nonventilated alveoli?

1. Compare the following two patients. Both are breathing room air.

Patient A		Patient B	
PaO_2	60 mm Hg	PaO_2	90 mm Hg
$PaCO_2$	35 mm Hg	$PaCO_2$	38 mm Hg
pH	7.46	pH	7.42
SaO_2	90%	SaO_2	97%
Hb	15 g/dL	Hb	10 g/dL

A. Which patient has better oxygenation? Explain.

KEY CONCEPT QUESTIONS

*Instructions: Choose the **single** best answer for each multiple choice question.*

1. End-capillary blood leaving a normal alveolus that is adequately ventilated with atmospheric air has a P_ACO_2 equal to:
   A. 40 mm Hg
   B. 0 mm Hg
   C. 45 mm Hg
   D. Mixed venous PCO_2

2. Arterial PO_2 is determined by the:
   A. Average of all end-capillary PO_2s
   B. Basal end-capillary O_2 contents
   C. Average of alveolar PO_2
   D. Average of all end-capillary O_2 contents

3. Major V/Q imbalance mechanisms causing hypoxemia include all of the following *except:*
   A. Overall hypoventilation
   B. Absolute dead space
   C. $\dot{V}/\dot{Q}$ mismatch
   D. Absolute shunt

4. Increasing the FiO_2 in patients with $\dot{V}/\dot{Q}$ mismatch will have which of the following effects?
   A. It will not improve PaO_2
   B. It will decrease PaO_2
   C. It will improve PaO_2
   D. It will increase $PaCO_2$

13 Clinical Assessment of Acid-Base and Oxygenation Status

OBJECTIVES

After reading this chapter, you will be able to:

- Differentiate between arterial blood gas classification and interpretation.
- Apply a systematic arterial blood gas classification method.
- Differentiate between oxygenation and ventilation defects.
- Explain the basis for compensatory activity in all acid-base disturbances.
- Indentify how the anion gap computation can help the clinician differentiate the causes of metabolic acidosis.
- Explain why acute changes in $PaCO_2$ affect the plasma $[HCO_3^-]$.
- Explain how acid-base disturbances affect plasma $[K^+]$ and $[Cl^-]$.
- Identify why the standard bicarbonate and base excess measurements more accurately reflect purely metabolic acid-base disturbances than plasma $[HCO_3^-]$.
- Differentiate between the traditional Henderson-Hasselbalch approach and Stewart's strong ion approach to acid-base physiology.
- Distinguish between pulmonary and cardiovascular factors that affect tissue oxygenation.
- Classify the causes of and the severity of oxygenation defects.
- Interpret various pulmonary and cardiovascular tissue oxygenation indicators.

KEY TERMS AND DEFINITIONS

Define the following terms:

1. Hypercapnia

2. Hypocapnia

3. Respiratory acidosis

4. Respiratory alkalosis

5. Metabolic acidosis

6. Metabolic alkalosis

7. Anion gap

8. Kussmaul's respiration

9. Standard bicarbonate

10. Base excess (BE)

11. Strong ion

12. Hypoxic hypoxia

13. Anemic hypoxia

14. Stagnant hypoxia

15. Histotoxic hypoxia

MATCHING

Match the following conditions with their associated acid-base disorder.

_____ 1. Hyperventilation

_____ 2. Prolonged vomiting

_____ 3. Hypoventilation

_____ 4. Prolonged diarrhea

_____ 5. Diabetic ketoacidosis

_____ 6. Arterial hypoxemia

_____ 7. Nasogastric drainage

_____ 8. Acute exacerbation of advanced COPD

A. Respiratory acidosis
B. Respiratory alkalosis
C. Metabolic acidosis
D. Metabolic alkalosis

Match each of the following blood gases to the statement that correctly identifies the degree of compensation.

_____ 1. pH = 7.25 $PaCO_2$ = 55 [HCO_3^-] = 24 mEq/L

_____ 2. pH = 7.42 $PaCO_2$ = 48 mm Hg [HCO_3^-] = 30 mEq/L

_____ 3. pH = 7.48 $PaCO_2$ = 50 mm Hg [HCO_3^-] = 29 mEq/L

A. Fully compensated
B. Partially compensated
C. Uncompensated

SHORT ANSWER/CRITICAL THINKING QUESTIONS

For questions 1 through 4, choose the correct answer from the choices offered in parentheses.

1. If arterial pH is 7.48, $PaCO_2$ is 42 mm Hg, and $[HCO_3^-]$ is 30 mEq/L, then (**acidemia, alkalemia, normal pH**) is present, the causative component is (**$PaCO_2$, $[HCO_3^-]$**), the compensating component is (**$PaCO_2$, $[HCO_3^-]$**), and this blood gas is classified as *uncompensated metabolic alkalosis.*

2. If arterial pH is 7.37, $PaCO_2$ is 48 mm Hg, and $[HCO_3^-]$ is 27 mEq/L, then (**acidemia, alkalemia, normal pH**) is present, pH is on the (**acidotic, alkalotic**) side of normal, this represents a (**noncompensated, compensated, partially compensated**) condition, the compensating component is (**$PaCO_2$, $[HCO_3^-]$**) and this blood gas is classified as *compensated respiratory acidosis.*

3. If arterial pH is 7.32, $PaCO_2$ is 30 mm Hg, and $[HCO_3^-]$ is 15 mEq/L, then (**acidemia, alkalemia, normal pH**) is present, the causative component is (**$PaCO_2$, $[HCO_3^-]$**), the compensating component is (**$PaCO_2$, $[HCO_3^-]$**), and the pH is (**noncompensated, compensated, partially compensated**).

4. If arterial pH is 7.47, $PaCO_2$ is 30 mm Hg, and $[HCO_3^-]$ is 21 mEq/L, then (**acidemia, alkalemia, normal pH**) is present, the causative component is (**$PaCO_2$, $[HCO_3^-]$**), the compensating component is (**$PaCO_2$, $[HCO_3^-]$**), and this blood gas is classified as (**noncompensated, compensated, partially compensated**).

103

Copyright © 2013 by Mosby, an imprint of Elsevier Inc. All rights reserved.

Chapter **13** Clinical Assessment of Acid-Base and Oxygenation Status

For questions 5 through 10, classify the following acid-base disorders using the four-step systematic approach outlined in the textbook.

5. pH = 7.16, PCO_2 = 75 mm Hg, $[HCO_3^-]$ = 26 mEq/L

6. pH = 7.33, PCO_2 = 60 mm Hg, $[HCO_3^-]$ = 31 mEq/L

7. pH = 7.47, PCO_2 = 48 mm Hg, $[HCO_3^-]$ = 34 mEq/L

8. pH = 7.27, PCO_2 = 36 mm Hg, $[HCO_3^-]$ = 16 mEq/L

9. pH = 7.48, PCO_2 = 33 mm Hg, $[HCO_3^-]$ = 24 mEq/L

Chapter **13**   **Clinical Assessment of Acid-Base and Oxygenation Status**

10. pH = 7.44, PCO_2 = 48 mm Hg, $[HCO_3^-]$ = 31 mEq/L

11. A COPD patient with a history of chronic CO_2 retention comes into the emergency room with hypoxemia and respiratory distress. A room air arterial blood gas shows:

   pH = 7.37
   PCO_2 = 55 mm Hg
   HCO_3 = 31
   PO_2 = 51
   SpO_2 = 82%

   Interpret this blood gas, including the patient's oxygenation status.

   Days later, the same patient develops a respiratory infection and presents with the following arterial blood gas results:

   pH = 7.43
   PCO_2 = 48 mm Hg
   HCO_3 = 31
   PO_2 = 45
   SpO_2 = 78%

   Interpret this blood gas, including the patient's oxygenation status.

12. A patient has the following blood gas:

   pH = 7.20, PCO_2 = 36 mm Hg, $[HCO_3^-]$ = 16 mEq/L
   This patient also has an "anion gap" of 23 mEq/L.
   A. What is the cause of an "anion gap?"

105

B. Give an example of a disease or condition consistent with this situation.

13. When a loss of bicarbonate induces an acidosis, another anion is gained via renal reabsorption, keeping the anion gap within normal limits. Identify this anion.

14. Which of these conditions would be associated with an anion gap? Explain.
    (a) extremely low blood pressure causing tissue hypoxia, (b) diabetes, (c) severe diarrhea.

15. Metabolic alkalosis may be caused by a gain of buffer base or a loss of fixed acids. Both of these causes produce a high plasma bicarbonate concentration. Explain why a loss of hydrogen ions (from fixed acids) causes the plasma bicarbonate to increase.

16. A. What types of chloride ion (Cl^-) and potassium ion (K^+) ion imbalance may cause metabolic alkalosis?

B. Briefly explain the mechanism involved.

17. A. What is the body's compensatory response to metabolic alkalosis?

B. What could limit this response, and what would be the result of this limitation?

18. Circle the correct responses in the following statement, or fill in the blank. An acute rise in $PaCO_2$ causes the $[HCO_3^-]$ to rise slightly (1 mEq/L per 10 mm Hg PCO_2 rise.) Thus, the plasma bicarbonate concentration is not a *pure* index of metabolic acid-base disturbances. However, if a patient's arterial blood sample is brought to the laboratory and first equilibrated to a gas with a PCO_2 of 40 mm Hg and *then* the bicarbonate concentration is measured, any abnormality in the $[HCO_3^-]$ must now be a reflection of a pure (**respiratory/metabolic**) acid-base

disturbance. This measurement of bicarbonate concentration is known as the _____.
Even this measurement has shortcomings as a purely metabolic index because the lab (*in vitro*) measurement has important differences compared to what actually would happen in the blood vessels (*in vivo measurement*) when plasma PCO_2 changes. Explain this difference and why the *in vitro* lab process introduces error.

19. A. Give an example of each type of hypoxia (anemic, hypoxic, stagnant, and histotoxic).

B. Identify which types of hypoxia do not benefit from the delivery of supplemental oxygen and why they do not benefit.

20. A. Calculate your normal predicted PaO_2 at sea level while in the standing position.

    B. Calculate the PaO_2 of an 82-year-old under the same conditions.

21. Fill in the blanks with the correct answers to complete the following statement:

    The PO_2 of a dry gas composed of 100% oxygen at sea level is _____ mm Hg.

    Therefore, at sea level, 1% oxygen represents a PO_2 of _____ mm Hg, and raising

    the FIO_2 by 0.1 (10%) raises the inspired PO_2 by _____ mm Hg. This translates to

    an alveolar PO_2 increase of about _____ mm Hg. If the $P(A-a)O_2$ is 10 mm Hg, this

    translates to an arterial PO_2 of about _____ mm Hg for every 10% increase in inspired

    oxygen concentration.

22. In Denver, the barometric pressure is about 633 mm Hg. The normal PaO_2 you calculated in #20B would change

    to _____ mm Hg in Denver.

1. An elderly asthmatic patient is brought to the clinic in acute respiratory distress. She has had the gastrointestinal "flu" for 2 days and indicates she has had diarrhea since her symptoms began. She is wheezing audibly, is very short of breath, and speaks in broken sentences. She now states that she ran out of her bronchodilator medication 3 days ago. An arterial blood gas performed while the patient was breathing room air reveals a PO_2 of 55 mm Hg, PCO_2 of 47 mm Hg, a pH of 7.25 and an $[HCO_3^-]$ of 20 mEq/L. A repeat blood gas after supplemental oxygen is given at 2 L/min by nasal cannula shows that the PO_2 has improved to 90 mm Hg.

   A. Classify the patient's acid-base disturbance and its cause.

   B. Identify the ventilation defect responsible for the low PO_2.

   C. What therapies will immediately address her acid-base and oxygenation problems?

2. Compare the following two patients. Both are breathing room air.

	Patient A	Patient B
PaO_2	48	95
$PaCO_2$	33	39
pH	7.48	7.33
HCO_3^-	24	20
SaO_2	83%	97%
Hb	15	15
CaO_2	16.8	19.8
$P(A-a)O_2$	52	5
Q_T	5.8	2.9
SvO_2	70%	50%
PvO_2	38	26
CvO_2	14.2	10.1

A. Which patient has impaired oxygen transfer in the lung? Explain.

B. Which patient has better tissue oxygenation? Explain and justify with evidence.

KEY CONCEPT QUESTIONS

*Choose the **single** best answer for each multiple choice question.*

1. Metabolic acidosis is associated with which of the following:
   A. Vomiting
   B. Diarrhea
   C. Nasogastric suction
   D. Diuretic therapy

2. Renal compensation for respiratory acidosis begins as soon as $PaCO_2$ rises. How long will it be before full compensation can be expected?
   A. 2 hours
   B. 8 hours
   C. 12 hours
   D. Several days

3. The abnormal acid-base condition produced by overly aggressive mechanical ventilation is called:
   A. Metabolic acidosis
   B. Metabolic alkalosis
   C. Respiratory alkalosis
   D. Respiratory acidosis

4. A general "rule of thumb" is that at sea level, an additional 10% F_IO_2 will increase PaO_2 by approximately:
   A. 10 mm Hg
   B. 50 mm Hg
   C. 47 mm Hg
   D. 76 mm Hg

Physiologic Basis for Advanced Oxygenation and Lung Protective Strategies

14

OBJECTIVES

After reading this chapter, you will be able to:

- Explain why monitoring $PaCO_2$ is an important consideration when monitoring oxygen therapy in patients with chronically hypercapnic chronic obstructive pulmonary disease (COPD).
- Identify why a change in body position might improve oxygenation in unilateral lung disease.
- Explain how various inflammatory processes injure the alveolar capillary membrane and produce severe shunting and hypoxemia in patients with acute respiratory distress syndrome (ARDS).
- Explain how positive end-expiratory pressure (PEEP) and continuous positive airway pressure (CPAP) improve oxygenation in ARDS.
- Differentiate between PEEP and CPAP indications and mechanisms of action.
- Identify how the interplay between alveolar and intrapleural pressures determine lung volume in both spontaneous and mechanically induced ventilation.
- Identify why pressure and volume cannot function as independent variables in producing alveolar stretch injury.
- Explain how to clinically monitor alveolar pressure, and explain the rationale for its measurement.
- Describe the mechanisms whereby alveolar overdistension, atelectrauma, and biotrauma are involved in ventilator-induced lung injury (VILI) and how they can be prevented during mechanical ventilation.
- Explain why the accepted standard of care for mechanically ventilated patients with ARDS might require the development of hypercapnia and acidosis.
- Identify the mechanisms whereby prone positioning of mechanically ventilated patients with ARDS improves oxygenation and reduces VILI.
- Differentiate, both mechanically and functionally, between volume- and pressure-targeted mechanical ventilation.
- Identify which protective lung ventilation strategies have been shown conclusively to reduce mortality in patients with ARDS.

KEY TERMS AND DEFINITIONS

Define the following terms:

1. Heterogeneous disease

2. Homogeneous disease

3. Acute lung injury

4. Acute respiratory distress syndrome

5. Atelectrauma

6. Biotrauma

7. Cytokines

8. Multisystem organ dysfunction syndrome (MODS)

9. Permissive hypercapnia

10. Prostaglandins

11. Retinopathy of prematurity (ROP)

12. Ventilator-induced lung injury (VILI)

13. Volutrauma

MATCHING

Match the terms below to the correct definition.

_____ 1. APRV

_____ 2. BiPAP/Bilevel

_____ 3. CPAP

_____ 4. PEEP

_____ 5. HFOV

_____ 6. Volume-targeted ventilation

_____ 7. Pressure-targeted ventilation

A. A ventilatory mode that maintains a constant inspiratory pressure at the endotracheal tube for a preset time regardless of the volume delivered

B. Altering high and low levels of continuous positive airway pressure with high CPAP levels lasting longer than low CPAP levels

C. Airway pressure applied to the airway in conjunction with endotracheal intubation and mechanical ventilation in which the airway pressure provided remains above atmospheric levels at the end of expiration

D. A ventilatory mode that is designed to cycle into expiration upon delivery of a preselected volume at a preselected flow rate

E. Airway pressure applied to a spontaneously breathing patient where a relatively constant positive airway pressure is maintained throughout inspiration and expiration

F. Alternating high and low levels of CPAP where high and low CPAP levels are applied for equal time periods or low CPAP time is longer than high CPAP duration

G. A type of mechanical ventilation that employs very high respiratory rates at very small tidal volumes

SHORT ANSWER/CRITICAL THINKING QUESTIONS

1. Explain why monitoring $PaCO_2$ is an important consideration when monitoring oxygen therapy in chronically hypercapnic COPD patients.

2. Explain why a supine position may *improve* arterial PO_2 in patients with hypovolemic shock (low blood volume and blood pressure), but may *decrease* PaO_2 in patients with congestive heart failure (a condition in which the ventricle's contractility is abnormally low, causing "pump" failure).

3. By what mechanism does PEEP or CPAP (1) improve lung compliance, and (2) reduce shunting and improve the arterial PO_2?

4. High inspiratory pressures and PEEP levels during mechanical ventilation may over-stretch and damage alveoli. By monitoring peak *alveolar* pressure, we can limit the pressure to which alveoli are subjected. *Remember, peak alveolar pressure is not the same as peak airway pressure measured at the endotracheal tube, i.e. the pressure monitored by the gauge on the mechanical ventilator.*

   What ventilator pressure measurement can you make that will be equal to alveolar pressure?

Chapter **14** **Physiologic Basis for Advanced Oxygenation and Lung Protective Strategies**

5. Stiff, non-compliant lungs of the severely diseased patient may not inflate to "normal" tidal volumes if we limit alveolar pressure to what we believe is a "safe" level.

   A. What may be the undesired consequences of this kind of ventilation strategy (i.e. limiting the inspiratory pressure to a "safe" level)?

   B. Under what circumstances may it be justifiable to use such a ventilation strategy, even though these negative consequences may occur?

   C. What is the term commonly used to describe this ventilation strategy?

A 55-year-old male was admitted to a general surgical unit after surgery for a bowel obstruction. The surgical procedure involved extensive abdominal surgery to repair a perforated colon. During surgery his systolic blood pressure dropped to 70 mm Hg. Six units of packed red blood cells and 3 L of normal saline were administered intravenously to restore blood loss and circulating volume. Currently he is receiving 60% oxygen through an aerosol face mask. Vital signs are as follows:

Respiratory rate: 28 breaths/minute
Heart rate: 120 beats/minute
Temperature: 39° C
Breath sounds: bilateral fine basilar crackles
The most recent chest x-ray shows bilateral infiltrates.

Arterial blood gases are drawn with the following results:

$pH = 7.35$
$PaO_2 = 50$ mm Hg
$PaCO_2 = 27$
$HCO_3^- = 16$
$SaO_2 = 84\%$

A. Review Box 14-1 in the textbook. What condition most likely led to the development of ARDS in this patient?

B. Explain the pathophysiology of ARDS.

C. Explain how ARDS can lead to refractory hypoxemia?

Chapter **14** **Physiologic Basis for Advanced Oxygenation and Lung Protective Strategies**

D. What are the possible complications this patient is at risk of developing secondary to ARDS?

E. Based on the assessment data presented, what do you recommend to treat this patient's hypoxemia?

KEY CONCEPT QUESTIONS

*Instructions: Choose the **single** best answer for each multiple choice question.*

1. In which of the following conditions would oxygen therapy be ineffective?
   A. Hypoventilation
   B. $\dot{V}/\dot{Q}$ mismatch
   C. Absolute shunting
   D. Diffusion defects

2. To better match ventilation and blood flow, a patient with ARDS should be positioned:
   A. Prone
   B. Supine
   C. Diseased lung down
   D. Diseased lung up

3. The severity of hypoxemia necessary to make the diagnosis of ARDS is defined by the ratio of the partial pressure of oxygen in the patient's arterial blood (PaO_2) to the fraction of oxygen in the inspired air (F_IO_2) that is:
   A. Less than 300 mm Hg
   B. Less than 200 mm Hg
   C. Greater than 300 mm Hg
   D. Greater than 200 mm Hg

4. Which of the following strategies is considered the standard of care in preventing alveolar collapse?
   A. Low tidal volume
   B. High PEEP
   C. Open lung approach
   D. Permissive hypercapnia

15 Physiology of Sleep-Disordered Breathing

OBJECTIVES

After reading this chapter, you will be able to:

- Explain how the brain regulates sleeping and waking cycles through neurocontrolled chemical mediators.
- Identify why the upper airway anatomy plays such a major role in sleep-disordered breathing.
- Distinguish between the three stages of non-rapid eye movement sleep and rapid eye movement sleep.
- Identify the six major categories of sleep disorders and the specific classification for sleep-disordered breathing.
- Differentiate between obstructive sleep apnea, central sleep apnea, mixed sleep apnea, childhood sleep apnea, and sudden infant death syndrome.
- Explain the effects of sleep-disordered breathing on the cardiovascular system.
- Identify the mechanisms of central hemodynamic dysfunction due to sleep-disordered breathing.
- Diagnose sleep-disordered breathing through the use of the polysomnogram.
- Explain the physiologic treatment of sleep-disordered breathing using positive airway pressure, oral appliances, positional therapy, and airway enlargement.

KEY TERMS AND DEFINITIONS

Define the following terms:

1. Sleep-disordered breathing (SDB)

2. Polysomnogram (PSG)

3. Hypothalamus

4. Optic chiasm

5. Suprachiasmatic nucleus (SCN)

6. Circadian rhythm

7. Ventrolateral preoptic nucleus (VLPO)

8. Mallampati score

9. Retrognathia

10. Macroglossia

11. Electroencephalogram (EEG)

12. Alpha waves

13. Delta waves

14. Non-rapid eye movement (NREM)

15. Rapid eye movement (REM)

16. Electromyography (EMG)

17. Sleep architecture

18. Sleep histogram

19. Sleep hygiene

20. Dyssomnia

21. Obstructive sleep apnea (OSA)

22. Apnea

23. Hypopnea

24. Micrognathia

25. Apnea-hypopnea index (AHI)

26. Central sleep apnea (CSA)

27. Excessive daytime somnolence

28. Respiratory effort related arousals (RERA)

29. Sudden infant death syndrome (SIDS)

30. Mixed sleep apnea (MSA)

31. Montage

32. Prescriptive pressure

33. Mandibular advancement device (MAD)

34. Tongue retaining device (TRD)

35. Uvulopalatopharyngoplasty (UPPP)

36. Maxillomandibular advancement

37. Radio frequency tissue ablation

38. Nasal cycling

MATCHING

Match the stages of sleep with the respective characteristics of sleep.

_____ 1. Stage 1 NREM

_____ 2. Stage 2 NREM

_____ 3. Stage 3 and 4 NREM

_____ 4. REM stage

A. Deepest level of sleep; EEG displays delta waves, or slow-wave sleep.

B. EEG shows a reduction in activity between wakefulness and sleep; accounts for 5% to 10% of the total sleep cycle.

C. Active sleep associated with loss of core body temperature regulation; dreaming occurs that lasts 10 to 20 minutes.

D. EEG displays sharp spikes called "K-complexes" and "sleep spindles"; approximately 40% to 50% of the total sleep period is spent in this stage.

119

LABELING

Label the following polysomnographic representations with the appropriate sleep-disordered breathing pattern.

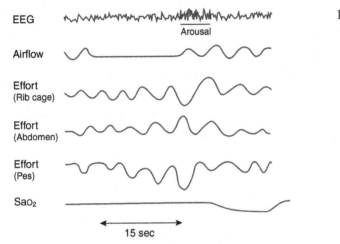

1. _____

(From Wilkins RL, et al: *Clinical assessment in respiratory care,* ed 6, St Louis, 2010, Mosby.)

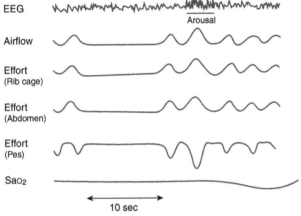

2. _____

(From Wilkins RL, et al: *Clinical assessment in respiratory care,* ed 6, St Louis, 2010, Mosby.)

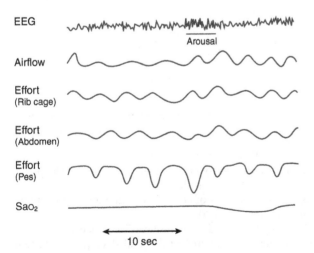

3. _____

(From Wilkins RL, et al: *Clinical assessment in respiratory care,* ed 6, St Louis, 2010, Mosby.)

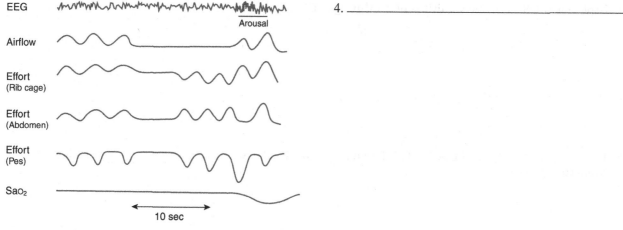

EEG

Arousal

Airflow

Effort
(Rib cage)

Effort
(Abdomen)

Effort
(Pes)

Sao₂

10 sec

4. _____

(From Wilkins RL, et al: *Clinical assessment in respiratory care,* ed 6, St Louis, 2010, Mosby.)

SHORT ANSWER/CRITICAL THINKING QUESTIONS

1. Explain how the onset of REM sleep causes arousals in patients with sleep-disordered breathing.

2. Explain the difference between hypopnea and respiratory effort related arousals (RERAs).

3. Explain how positive airway pressure devices correct airway obstruction in OSA.

4. What sleep breathing disorder requires the use of BiPAP? Explain.

Chapter **15** **Physiology of Sleep-Disordered Breathing**

5. Explain how OSA can affect activities of daily living (ADLs).

6. Define mixed sleep apnea (MSA); include how it is diagnosed and how treatment of MSA is different than treatment for OSA.

CASE STUDY

M.J., a 55-year-old male, presents to his primary care physician with the complaint of excessive daytime sleepiness and morning headaches. His wife states that he snores loudly and frequently quits breathing and gasps throughout the night. He states that he has difficulty concentrating at work and also has had episodes of dozing off while driving. He has a history of hypertension and smokes two packs of cigarettes a day. He consumes three to five cups of coffee per day and also drinks two to three beers in the evening. He does not exercise on a regular basis.

Physical Assessment:
Height: 5 ft, 11 in
Weight: 250 lb
RR: 24 breaths/min
HR: 122 beats/min
BP: 162/90
Neck size: 17.5 in
BMI: 34.9 lb/in^2

1. What aspects of the patient history are relevant to OSA?

2. What is the significance of the neck size and BMI?

Polysomnogram Results:

Total REM sleep	2% (normal 15%-20%)
Stage 1 NREM	8% (normal 5%-10%)
Stage 2 NREM	77% (normal 40%-50%)
Stage 3 NREM	13% (normal 25%)

There were 42 obstructive apneas, 6 central apneas, and 7 mixed apneas for a total of 55 apneic episodes in a 2-hour period. There were 260 hypopneas and the AHI was 157.5. There were 310 respiratory events with SpO_2 desaturations greater than 3%. The number of snores during sleep was 2112. The lowest SpO_2 was 60% and the mean SpO_2 during sleep was 85%. There were 200 periodic limb movements resulting in 14 arousals. The total arousal index was 83.4 per hour.

3. How would you interpret the polysomnogram results?

KEY CONCEPT QUESTIONS

Instructions: Choose the single best answer for each multiple choice question.

1. In which level of sleep is "restorative sleep" thought to occur?
   A. Stage 1 NREM
   B. Stage 2 NREM
   C. Stage 3 NREM
   D. REM

2. A 50% reduction in the tidal volume for at least 10 seconds during sleep defines which of the following?
   A. Apnea
   B. Sleep arousal
   C. Hypopnea
   D. RERA

3. Which breathing pattern is a common sign of central sleep apnea?
   A. Cheyne-Stokes respirations
   B. Kussmaul's respirations
   C. Biot's respirations
   D. Apneustic respirations

4. The lack of dreaming could mean that a patient is not spending a significant period of sleep in which stage?
   A. Stage 1 NREM
   B. Stage 2 NREM
   C. Stage 3 NREM
   D. REM

16 Fetal and Newborn Cardiopulmonary Physiology

OBJECTIVES

After reading this chapter, you will be able to:

- Identify what happens during each of the five stages of fetal lung development.
- Explain how prematurity might lead to respiratory failure in the newborn.
- Explain how gas exchange occurs between fetal and maternal blood.
- Describe how alterations in maternal-fetal physiology affect fetal development.
- Identify the key anatomic differences between infant and adult airways.
- Describe the physiologic responses to heat loss in the infant.
- Explain how the infant generates heat.
- Explain how the fetal cardiovascular system forms and becomes functional early in gestation.
- Identify what factors determine whether the fetus is viable for postnatal life.
- Identify the key anatomic and physiologic differences between fetal and neonatal circulation.
- Describe the key events that occur during transition from fetal to extrauterine life.
- Explain how acyanotic and cyanotic cardiac defects affect the neonate.

KEY TERMS AND DEFINITIONS

Define the following terms:

1. Abruptio placentae

2. Amniocentesis

3. Brown fat

4. Choanal atresia

5. Chorionic villi

6. Ductus arteriosus

7. Ductus venosus

8. Extracorporeal life support

9. Foramen ovale

10. Meconium

11. Neutral thermal environment

12. Oligohydramnios

13. Polyhydramnios

14. Teratogen

15. Wharton's jelly

FILL IN THE BLANK

Number the following statements describing fetal lung growth in the order in which they occur in the developing fetus. (Numbers 1-5)

_____ Type I and type II cells and immature surfactant are present.

_____ Mature surfactant is present.

_____ Mainstem bronchi are formed.

_____ Efficient gas exchange occurs across alveolar capillary membrane.

_____ Diaphragm development is complete.

MATCHING

Match the following statements with the stage of pulmonary development in which they occur. (Letters may be used more than once.)

_____ 1. Early alveoli development occurs.

_____ 2. Heart formation is complete.

_____ 3. Alveoli continue to increase in number and size.

_____ 4. Lung emerges as an outpouching of the fetal foregut.

_____ 5. Fetus is potentially capable of gas exchange.

_____ 6. Pulmonary arteries and veins begin to form.

_____ 7. Conducting airways are completed.

_____ 8. Cilia, mucous glands, goblet cells appear

_____ 9. Segmental bronchi are formed.

_____ 10. Pulmonary capillary development begins.

A. Embryonic period (Day 26 to Week 6)
B. Pseudoglandular period (Weeks 7-16)
C. Canalicular period (Weeks 17-26)
D. Saccular period (Weeks 26-36)
E. Alveolar period (Week 36 to 2 years)

Congenital Cardiac Defects

Match the descriptions on the right to the appropriate figure on the left.

_____ 1.

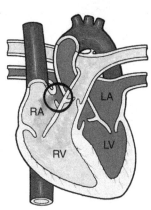

_____ 2.

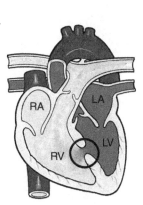

_____ 3.

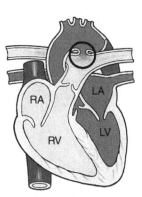

_____ 4.

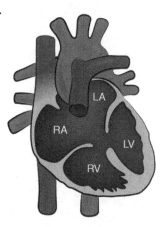

A. Ventricular septal defect
B. Atrioventricular septal defect
C. Anomalous venous return
D. Atrial septal defect
E. Truncus arteriosus
F. Hypoplastic left heart
G. Transposition of the great arteries
H. Coarctation of the aorta
I. Tetralogy of Fallot
J. Patent ductus arteriosus
K. Aortic stenosis
L. Tricuspid atresia

_____ 5.

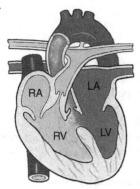

_____ 6.

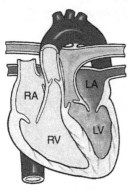

_____ 7.

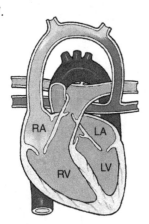

_____ 8.

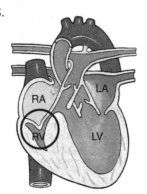

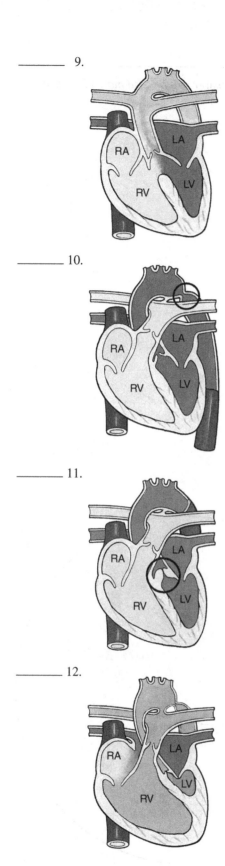

_____ 9.

_____ 10.

_____ 11.

_____ 12.

Label the following structures of the placenta and developing fetus. The same answer will be used more than once.

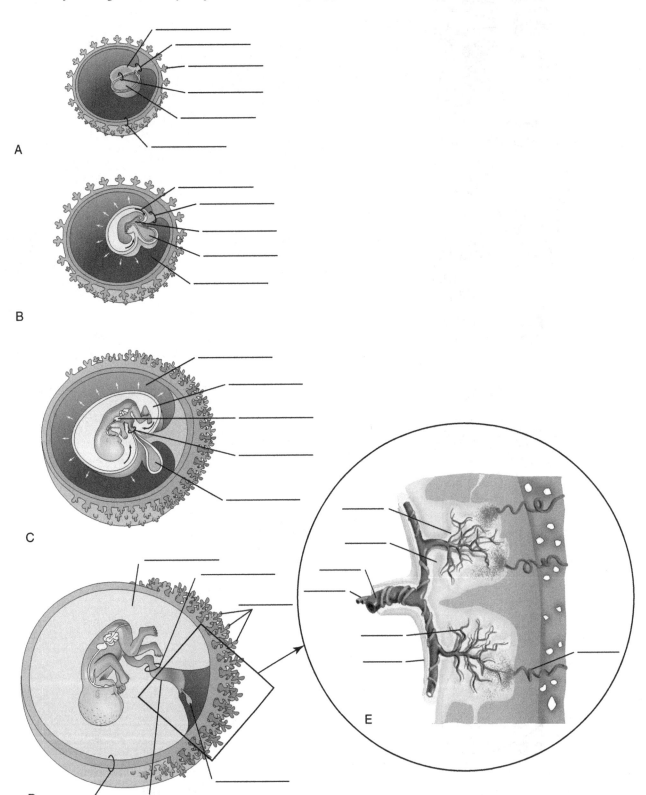

(**A-D,** From Moore KL: The developing human: clinically oriented embryology, ed 8, Philadelphia, 2008, Saunders; **E,** From Wilkins RL, et al, editors: *Fundamentals of respiratory care,* ed 8, St Louis, 2003, Mosby.)

Label the structures and organs associated with fetal circulation:

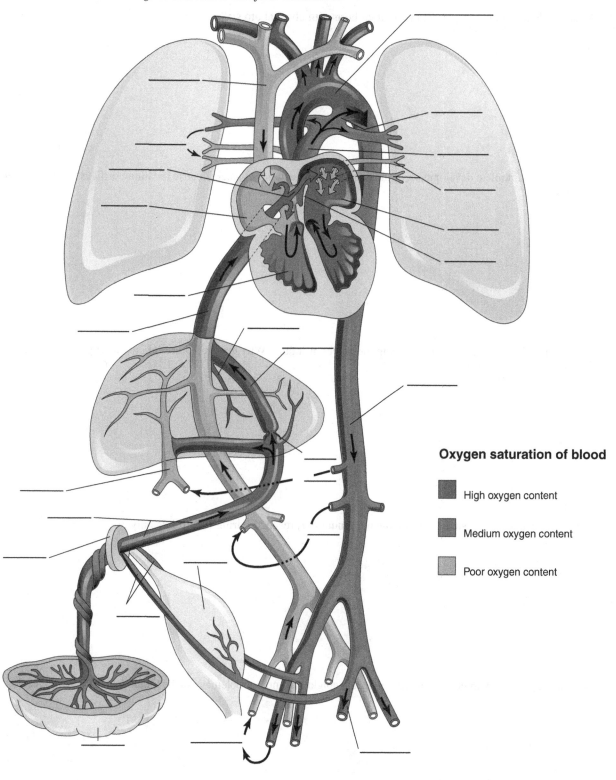

Oxygen saturation of blood

■ High oxygen content

■ Medium oxygen content

□ Poor oxygen content

1. What problems would you expect in an infant born with choanal atresia?

2. How would incomplete development of the diaphragm in gestational week 7 cause breathing difficulties in an infant after birth?

3. What factors lead to increased heat loss in the newborn infant? Why are premature infants more prone to heat loss than term infants?

4. Explain how a fetus can survive, when the maximum PO_2 reached during fetal life is only 30 mm Hg.

5. Why are upper airway infections such as croup and epiglottitis more problematic in the infant than they are in the adult?

6. Why is the heart the first organ system to develop and function in the fetus?

7. Describe blood flow through the three fetal shunts.

8. Describe the respiratory transition to extrauterine life.

9. Describe circulatory changes that occur at birth and the resultant closure of the fetal shunts.

10. Use the APGAR score to assess the following neonatal condition. What treatment is indicated?
    Following a precipitous delivery (< 30 min) a 2400-gram infant is born by vaginal delivery. One minute after delivery the neonate has a heart rate of 100 and has good color except for some peripheral cyanosis. The baby grimaces in response to a suction catheter being placed into her nasal passages, but does not cry. She has some muscle tone but is not active. Respirations are slow and gasping.

Chapter **16** **Fetal and Newborn Cardiopulmonary Physiology**

11. The majority of congenital cardiac defects are classified as either *acyanotic* or *cyanotic*.

    A. Explain the difference between the two.

    B. What clinical findings would be present for each type of defect?

12. Patent ductus arteriosus can be classified as either a left-to-right shunt or a right-to-left shunt. Explain.

You are a respiratory therapist called to the neonatal intensive care unit (NICU) to be present at a high-risk delivery. Prior to delivery, you read through the mother's chart and learn the following:

This is the second pregnancy for this 38-year-old mother. Her first child was delivered at 32 weeks, due to premature rupture of the amniotic membranes associated with polyhydramnios, and was treated in the NICU for mild respiratory distress syndrome (RDS).

This pregnancy has been difficult, and the mother has been on bed rest for the last 8 weeks due to *placenta previa* (abnormally low implantation of the placenta in the uterus).

One hour ago the mother noticed some cramping and vaginal bleeding, leading to the decision to proceed to delivery to avoid further complications to mother and baby. The physician suspects *abruptio placentae* is the cause of the vaginal bleeding. Gestational age of the fetus is estimated to be 30 weeks.

A. What factors in the history given above are associated withan increased need for neonatal resuscitation?

Baby boy Andrew is delivered via cesarean section delivery 30 minutes later and is noted to be cyanotic and meconium stained. His 1-minute and 5-minute APGAR scores are 2 and 3, respectively. He is currently being resuscitated with bag mask ventilation and cardiac compressions are delivered at >100 per minute. An arterial blood gas obtained from the umbilical artery after the cord was cut reveals a pH of 7.22. The neonatologist is preparing to intubate baby boy Andrew and administer surfactant.

B. What factors surrounding this delivery are associated with increased risk of cardiopulmonary complications to baby boy Andrew?

Following intubation, surfactant is administered to baby boy Andrew and he is placed on mechanical ventilation. Two hours later, baby boy Andrew's oxygen needs increase and he develops increased respiratory distress. The neonatologist suspects persistent pulmonary hypertension of the newborn (PPHN) and orders inhaled nitric oxide therapy.

C. Why was surfactant administered to baby boy Andrew? Was the surfactant treatment successful?

D. Describe the use of nitric oxide therapy in the treatment of PPHN.

Instructions: Choose the **single** best answer for each multiple choice question.

1. When is alveolar development complete?
   A. Canalicular period
   B. Saccular period
   C. Alveolar period
   D. Age 8

2. Which of the following may contribute to difficult breathing in an infant?
   A. Small nose and mouth
   B. Large tongue
   C. Smaller airways
   D. Shorter, less stable trachea
   E. All of the above

3. What percentage of the blood in the pulmonary artery enters the pulmonary circulation to perfuse the fetal lung?
   A. 10%
   B. 30%
   C. 50%
   D. 70%

4. Which of the following conditions could delay the closure of the ductus arteriosus?
   A. Hypoglycemia
   B. Hyperthermia
   C. Hypoxia
   D. Hyperoxemia

17 Functional Anatomy of the Cardiovascular System

OBJECTIVES

After reading this chapter, you will be able to:

- Identify the gross anatomy and function of each of the heart's structures.
- Explain how the atria, ventricles, and heart valves work together to pump blood through the pulmonary and systemic circulations.
- Explain why the heart muscle is more blood flow dependent for oxygenation than other muscles in the body.
- Identify why extremely high heart rates can result in low cardiac stroke volumes and coronary artery blood flow.
- Explain how the specialized cardiac conduction system coordinates the synchronized contraction and relaxation of the atria and ventricles.
- Explain how cellular mechanisms, calcium ions, and adenosine triphosphate work together to bring about myocardial contraction and relaxation.
- Describe how the Frank-Starling mechanism helps the heart adjust to pump-varying amounts of blood.
- Explain the timing and sequence of all mechanical events in the cardiac cycle.
- Explain how pumping action and arterial elasticity work together to produce continuous blood flow.
- Identify how different mechanisms work to control the distribution of blood flow through systemic capillary beds.
- Explain why high diastolic pressure is more indicative of increased vascular resistance than is high systolic pressure.
- Explain why independent right ventricular pumping failure produces a different type of circulatory derangement than does left ventricular failure.
- Identify how local, central, and humoral mechanisms regulate blood pressure.

KEY TERMS AND DEFINITIONS

Define the following terms:

1. Point of maximum impulse

2. Pericardium

3. Epicardium

4. Myocardium

5. Endocardium

6. Tricuspid valve

7. Bicuspid valve

8. Pulmonary semilunar valve

9. Aortic semilunar valve

10. Chordae tendineae

11. Angina pectoris

12. Myocardial infarction

13. Sinoatrial node (SA node)

14. Atrioventricular node (AV node)

15. Bundle of His

16. Purkinje's fibers

17. Frank-Starling mechanism

18. Preload

19. Afterload

20. Stroke volume

21. Pulse pressure

22. Mean arterial pressure

23. Systemic vascular resistance

FILL IN THE BLANK

1. Number the following structures sequentially (1-13), in the order that blood flows through them from the systemic venous side of the heart.

   _____ Left ventricle

   _____ Right ventricle

   _____ Left atrium

   _____ Right atrium

   _____ Pulmonic valve

   _____ Tricuspid valve

   _____ Aortic valve

   _____ Bicuspid valve

   _____ Superior and inferior vena cava

   _____ Pulmonary artery

   _____ Aorta

   _____ Lungs

   _____ Pulmonary veins

2. Number the following events (1-10) in the cardiac cycle. The start point has been identified by the number 1.

   _____ Ventricular pressures rise enough to open semilunar valves.

   _____ The ventricles contract against closed semilunar valves.

   ___1___ Ventricular pressures build, forcefully closing the atrioventricular valves.

   _____ Atrial pressures fall as blood drains into the ventricles.

   _____ Back flow of blood into ventricles is stopped abruptly, causing dilation and recoil of the aorta and pulmonary artery.

   _____ The ventricles relax: their pressures fall, and the semilunar valves snap shut.

139

_____ Ventricular contraction closes the atrioventricular valves.

_____ The ejection period occurs.

_____ The atria contract, slightly distending ventricular walls.

_____ Ventricular pressures fall and atrioventricular valves open.

MATCHING

Match the anatomic terms below with their appropriate description:

_____ Trabeculae carneae

_____ Chordae tendineae

_____ Myocardium

_____ Foramen ovale

_____ Papillary muscles

_____ Fibrous annuli

_____ Pericardial fluid

_____ Visceral pericardium

A. Epicardium
B. Forms the bulk of the heart wall
C. Muscle bundles on the ventricular inner surface
D. Allows frictionless cardiac movement
E. Cone-shaped pillars
F. Tethers that prevent atrioventricular valvular regurgitation
G. Small depression in the interatrial septum
H. Connected ring framework to which muscle and valves are attached

LABELING

Label the features of the cardiac conduction system on the illustration below: AV node, SA node, internodal bundles, AV bundle, Interatrial bundle, Purkinje fibers, Right and left branches of the AV bundle, Septum, Lateral ventricular wall, RA, LA, RV, LV.

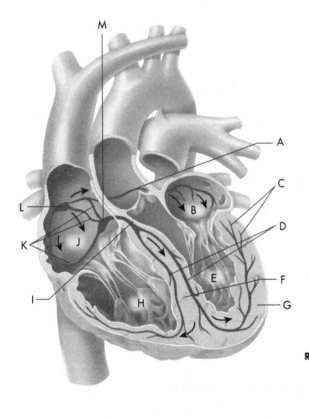

A. _____

B. _____

C. _____

D. _____

E. _____

F. _____

G. _____

H. _____

I. _____

J. _____

K. _____

L. _____

M. _____

(From Patton KT, Thibodeau GA: _Anatomy & physiology_, ed 7, St Louis, 2010, Mosby.)

1. Name the three layers of tissue that form the heart's ventricular walls in order from the most outer layer to the most inner layer.

2. Where are the *trabeculae carneae* located, and what is their purpose?

3. What are the consequences of a small opening in the ventricular septum?

4. Describe the cardiac skeleton.

5. Discuss the consequences of tricuspid regurgitation, including signs and symptoms.

6. Discuss the consequences of pulmonary semilunar valve stenosis, including signs and symptoms.

7. Why might a very high heart rate result in:
   A. A small stroke volume

   B. Reduced coronary artery blood flow.

8. What is the physiologic benefit of the AV node's decreased impulse conduction velocity?

9. Describe the structure of the T-tubule and the "triad" composed of T-tubules and sarcoplasmic reticulum. In your description, name the ions that are stored in the T-tubules and their effect on muscle contraction.

10. Explain the sequence of events occurring during muscle contraction (excitation and contraction) and include a description of cross-bridge formation.

11. Explain the physiology behind the Frank-Starling law as follows:
    A. Why does stretching the myocardial fiber increase the force of contraction?

    B. Why does overstretching the fiber or maximally shortening the fiber decrease the force of contraction?

12. Define the term *preload*. How is it measured in the clinical setting?

13. Discuss the following in terms of which is longer and roughly by how much.
    A. Ventricular ejection versus ventricular filling time

B. Ventricular passive filling (no atrial contraction) versus active filling (atrial contraction)

14. What is the normal stroke volume (in milliliters) compared to normal end-diastolic volume (in each ventricle)?

15. Your patient has a left ventricular ejection fraction of 45%.
    A. How does this compare to a normal ejection fraction?

    B. What does this suggest about the patient's cardiac function?

    C. What could cause this problem?

16. Which of the following is the most accurate statement? *(Circle the correct response.)*

    A. The heart dictates how much blood is ejected into the aorta with each stroke.

    B. The venous blood flowing into the heart dictates how much blood the heart must eject with each stroke.

17. Besides pressure generated by ventricular contraction, what other force continues to propel blood through the tissue capillary beds during ventricular diastole?

18. Why do abnormally stiff arteries cause the difference between systolic and diastolic pressures (pulse pressure) to increase?

19. Systolic pressure depends primarily on stroke volume ejected and arterial vessel recoil. Diastolic pressure depends mainly on peripheral vascular resistance. Explain why this is true.

20. Regarding mean arterial pressure:

    A. Why is it not accurate to take an average of the systolic and diastolic pressure to represent the mean arterial pressure?

    B. What formula can be used to estimate mean arterial pressure?

145

You are caring for a patient with chronic obstructive pulmonary disease who was admitted to the intensive care unit for a severe exacerbation of his pulmonary disease. A Swan-Ganz catheter has been placed in the patient's pulmonary artery to monitor hemodynamic status. The patient currently exhibits pedal edema and jugular venous distension (JVD). Central venous pressure (CVP) is 16 mm Hg. Reviewing the patient's chart, you notice that the patient's home medications include a dose of furosemide, a diuretic. The patient's current hospital medication list does not include any drugs with diuretic effects. You also note a weight gain of 2 kilograms (4.4 pounds) since admission yesterday. Your patient's oxygenation status demonstrates continued hypoxia due to the current exacerbation. You contact the intensivist to ask that the patient's diuretic medication be restarted.

A. What reasons will you give for adding it to his hospital medication list?

B. What is the cause of this patient's right heart failure?

KEY CONCEPT QUESTIONS

*Choose the **single** best answer for each multiple choice question.*

1. Coronary arteries receive blood directly from the:
   A. Left ventricle
   B. Aorta
   C. Pulmonary trunk
   D. Left atrium

2. Myocardial ischemia is the direct result of:
   A. Myocardial tissue death
   B. Angina pectoris
   C. Coronary artery occlusion
   D. Coronary artery vasodilation

3. Electrical impulses that stimulate ventricular contraction are initiated by the:
   A. SA node
   B. AV node
   C. Purkinje's fibers
   D. Intranodal pathway

4. Venous blood flow increases in the presence of:
   A. Arterial vasodilation
   B. Decreased blood volume
   C. Increased right atrial pressures (CVP)
   D. Decreased venous tone

18 Cardiac Electrophysiology

After reading this chapter, you will be able to:

- Explain the physiologic significance of the cardiac fiber's resting membrane potential (RMP) and how it is established.
- Identify how the relationship between the cardiac fiber's RMP and threshold potential affects the fiber's tendency to depolarize.
- Identify why depolarization of the cardiac fiber causes the fiber to contract.
- Explain the nature of the electrochemical events that cause the cardiac muscle fiber to spontaneously depolarize.
- Identify the mechanism whereby electrical charge differences across the cardiac cell membrane affect its permeability to Na^+, K^+, and Ca^{++} ions.
- Identify why abnormalities in blood Ca^{++} and K^+ concentrations affect cardiac muscle depolarization.
- Correlate the activity of ion channels and gates with the graphical voltage versus time representation (action potential) of a single cardiac fiber's depolarization and repolarization.
- Explain why catecholamine drugs increase cardiac contractility.
- Identify why calcium channel–blocking drugs affect heart muscle contractility.
- Describe the mechanisms whereby various drugs affect cardiac contractility and excitability.
- Explain how ectopic foci arising from (1) increased tissue excitability and (2) the sinoatrial (SA) nodal block differ from each other.
- Identify the purpose of the impulse transmission delay between the SA node and ventricles.
- Explain what happens when atrial impulses are blocked and prevented from entering the ventricles.
- Identify how sympathetic and parasympathetic stimulation affects heart muscle automaticity, rhythmicity, and excitability.

KEY TERMS AND DEFINITIONS

Define the following terms:

1. Resting membrane potential

2. Sodium-potassium exchange pump

3. Action potential

4. Threshold potential

5. Depolarization

6. Repolarization

7. Refractory

8. Excitability

9. Inotropic

10. Hypokalemia

11. Hyperkalemia

12. Catecholamine

13. Automaticity

14. SA node

15. Ectopic foci

16. Overdrive suppression

17. Downward displacement of the pacemaker

18. Bachmann bundle

19. AV bundle

20. Purkinje system conduction

MATCHING

Match the letter of the statement that correctly defines the following terms:

_____ Depolarization

_____ Repolarization

_____ Action potential

_____ Threshold potential

_____ Excitability

_____ Hyperpolarized

_____ Refractory

A. Difference between resting membrane and threshold potentials

B. Resting membrane potential changes to 0 millivolts (mV).

C. All activation gates open, allowing rapid influx of Na^+

D. Resting membrane potential changes to –90 mV

E. Cardiac muscle fiber unresponsive to stimuli during action potential phases 0-3

F. Cardiac cell membrane less susceptible to depolarization

G. The change in cardiac cell membrane potential as the cardiac fiber depolarizes and repolarizes

Match the letter of each statement to the correct ion involved in cardiac conduction. You will use more than one letter to describe each ion.

_____ Sodium (Na⁺)

_____ Potassium (K⁺)

_____ Calcium (Ca⁺⁺)

A. Extracellular concentration = 4 mEq/L
B. Three of these ions are pumped out of the cell for every two K⁺ ions
C. Intracellular concentration = 151 mEq/L
D. Moves through slow channels to stimulate action potential
E. Moves through fast channels to stimulate action potential
F. Extracellular concentration = 144 mEq/L
G. Rapid influx of this ion into the cell stimulates depolarization
H. Intracellular concentration = 5 mEq/L
I. Moves out of the cell due to diffusion
J. Flows into cell during phase 2 of the action potential
K. Intracellular concentration = 7 mEq/L
L. Cardiac muscle contraction directly related to extracellular levels of this ion
M. High levels of this ion increase membrane excitability

LABELING

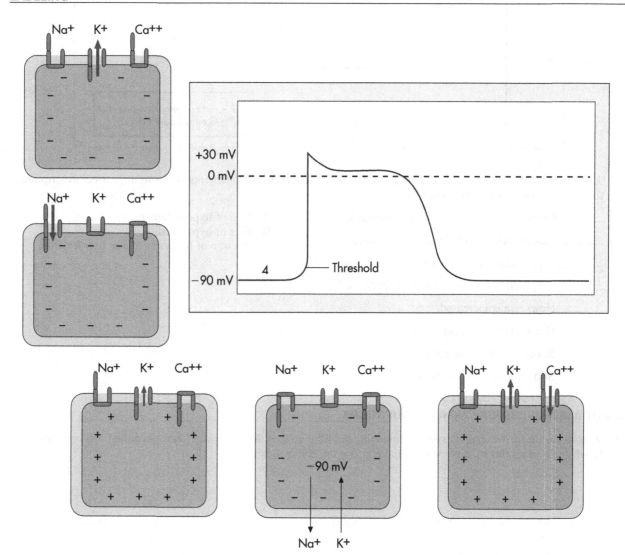

1. Correctly number the phases (0-4) of Na⁺, K⁺, and Ca⁺⁺ movement as they occur during generation of action potential in the above illustration. Then place the phase numbers in the appropriate position on the action potential waveform.

2. On the voltage-time graph below, draw the relative positions of three action potentials as they appear in normal, hypokalemic, and hyperkalemic conditions.

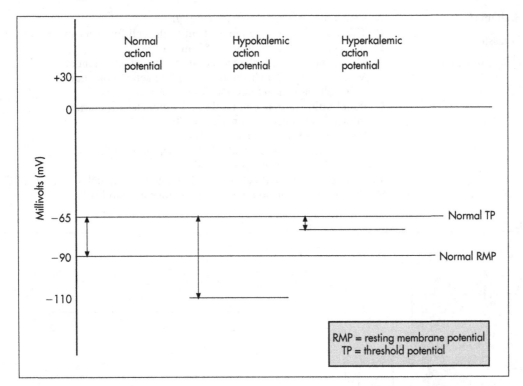

3. Use the completed diagram above to help you match the letters of the statements below to the correct description. You may use letters more than once.

_____ Cardiac cell membrane is more excitable.

_____ Cardiac cell membrane is less excitable.

_____ Amplitude of action potential is increased.

_____ Amplitude of action potential is decreased.

_____ Heart rate is increased.

_____ Heart rate is decreased.

_____ Stroke volume is increased.

_____ Stroke volume is decreased.

A. True of hyperkalemia
B. True of hypokalemia
C. Not true of hyperkalemia or hypokalemia

SHORT ANSWER/CRITICAL THINKING QUESTIONS

1. What is meant by the term *membrane potential*, and what creates this "potential" across cardiac cell membranes? In what way does this membrane potential *polarize* the cell membrane?

2. What determines the resting membrane potential (RMP)?

3. Is the cardiac cell membrane **polarized** or **depolarized** *(circle one)* when a muscle is relaxed? What electrical event initiates the activity responsible for cardiac muscle contraction?

4. The resting membrane potential (RMP) of myocardial cells is about −90 mV. This means that the muscle cell's interior is (**electropositive/electronegative**) *(circle one)* compared to the cell's exterior.

5. Explain the role of each of the following in creating the resting membrane potential (RMP):
   A. The K^+ concentration inside and outside of the cell, and which way K^+ diffuses.

   B. The high concentration of large, non-diffusible protein anions in the cell.

C. The sodium-potassium exchange pump.

6. What electrical changes cause the cardiac cell membrane Na$^+$ and K$^+$ channel gates to open or close?

7. What does the term *action potential* mean, and how is it recorded?

8. Describe the four phases of the action potential by identifying the electrical and chemical changes that occur in each stage.

9. The _____ channels are "fast" channels compared to the slower _____ channels. At what phase in the action potential does calcium enter the myocardial cell?

10. How does hyperkalemia cause the cardiac cell's resting membrane potential to become closer to its threshold potential? What are the clinical consequences?

11. How does hypokalemia cause the RMP to move farther away from the threshold threshold potential? What are the clinical consequences?

12. Explain the effects of hypocalcemia and hypercalcemia on myocardial excitability.

13. All myocardial fibers are capable of self-excitation or self-depolarization. This occurs because of a slow influx

    of _____ ions into the cell, which gradually raises the membrane potential to the level of the threshold potential (TP). A cardiac muscle fiber with an RMP of –55 mV and a TP of –45 mV will self-depolarize **(sooner/later)** *(circle one)* than a fiber with an RMP of –90 mV, and a TP of –70 mV.

14. Which cardiac muscle cells generate impulses with the greatest frequency? _____ Where is

    this tissue located? _____.
    Why do these cells have a greater firing rate than all other cardiac cells?

15. What causes a premature beat? What is another term used to describe a premature beat?

16. The inherent rate of firing (**increases/decreases**) *(circle one)* when moving downward from the atrial fibers toward ventricular fibers. Thus, if the AV bundle is blocked, the ventricular rate will be (**faster/slower**) *(circle one)* than the SA node rate.

17. Describe the impact of an abnormally high AV conduction rate on cardiac output.

18. Why are calcium channel blocker drugs used to treat patients with coronary artery disease?

CASE STUDIES

1. You are the respiratory therapist caring for a patient admitted to the hospital for treatment of an acute exacerbation of asthma. From the chart you learn that this patient also has a history of coronary artery disease. You will be administering a beta-agonist bronchodilator drug to relieve the patient's bronchospasm. What change in cardiac vital signs should be anticipated for this patient? What adverse effects could a beta-agonist bronchodilator cause in this patient?

2. Why should a calcium channel blocker not be given to a patient with very low blood pressure?

*Instructions: Choose the **single** best answer for each multiple choice question.*

1. The electrical event in the myocardial cell that leads to muscle fiber contraction is called:
   A. Resting membrane potential
   B. Threshold potential
   C. Voltage-sensitive activation gate
   D. Action potential

2. The main *intracellular* ion involved in generating the resting membrane potential is:
   A. Ca^{++}
   B. Cl^-
   C. K^+
   D. Na^+

3. Permeability of the myocardial cell membrane to Na^+ and K^+ is mainly controlled by:
   A. Voltage-sensitive gating proteins
   B. Leak channels
   C. Slow channels
   D. The sodium-potassium exchange pump

4. Which of the following may produce premature heart beats?
   A. Local areas of tissue hypoxia
   B. Mechanical irritation of the tissue
   C. Toxic irritation
   D. All of the above

19 The Electrocardiogram and Cardiac Arrhythmias in Adults

KEY TERMS AND DEFINITIONS

Define the following terms:

1. Electrocardiogram (ECG)

2. P wave

3. QRS complex

4. T wave

5. P-R interval

6. ST segment

7. Q-T interval

8. Relative refractory period

9. Bipolar leads

10. Unipolar leads

11. Precordial leads

12. Mean cardiac vector

13. Einthoven triangle

14. Tachycardia

15. Bradycardia

16. Fibrillation

17. Junctional rhythm

18. Pulse deficit

19. Bigeminy

20. Circus reentry

21. Defibrillation

MATCHING

Basic Rhythm Generation

Match components of the ECG on the left with the correct statement on the right. (Note: Each ECG component may have more than one correct statement, and some statements may not be used.)

_____ P wave

_____ QRS complex

_____ T wave

_____ P-R segment

_____ ST segment

_____ Q-T interval

A. Produced by ventricular repolarization
B. Produced by atrial depolarization
C. Represents ventricular refractory period
D. Represents time required for SA node impulse to travel to ventricles
E. Represents ventricular conduction time
F. Represents early phase of ventricular repolarization
G. Associated with ventricular contraction
H. Produced by atrial repolarization
I. Associated with ventricular relaxation
J. Associated with atrial contraction

ECG Abnormalities

Match each ECG abnormality on the left with the appropriate cardiac activity on the right.

_____ More P waves than QRS complexes

_____ P wave polarity opposite of expected change in
P wave size, shape, polarity

_____ Wide QRS complex

_____ Inverted, hidden, or retrograde P wave

_____ P-R interval greater than 0.2 sec

_____ Two QRS complexes of different polarity

A. Slowed SA node–ventricular impulse conduction
B. Not all atrial impulses are conducted to the ventricles
C. Slowed ventricular conduction velocity
D. Presence of ectopic focus
E. Impulse may originate in the AV node
F. Atrial pacemaker site has changed

Abnormal Rhythms

Choose the statement on the right that best describes the abnormal rhythm on the left.

_____ Atrial flutter

_____ Atrial fibrillation

_____ Junctional escape rhythm

_____ Premature ventricular contraction

_____ Junctional tachycardia

_____ Paroxysmal supraventricular tachycardia

A. Caused by an irritable ectopic focus in ventricular fibers
B. In the absence of SA node impulses, firing rate of
40-60/min
C. Caused by supraventricular pacemaker firing at
240-360/min
D. Junctional fibers generate a heart rate greater than
60 beats/min
E. Junctional fibers generate bursts of heart rates up to
240 beats/min
F. Uncoordinated discharge from ectopic atrial foci at a
rate of 300-600 beats/min

Abnormal Rhythms: Types of AV Conduction Block

Choose the statement on the right that best describes the type of heart block on the left. You may choose more than one descriptor for each type of AV conduction block.

_____ First-degree AV block

_____ Second-degree AV block (type I)

_____ Second-degree AV block (type II)

_____ Third degree AV block

A. P-R intervals gradually lengthen until QRS complex
fails to appear after P wave
B. No relationship between P waves and QRS complexes
C. Also known as Wenckebach's block
D. Constant P-R intervals with abnormal conduction ratios
E. P-R interval prolonged > 0.2 second
F. Also known as Mobitz type I block
G. Also known as complete heart block
H. Also known as Mobitz type II block

Chapter **19** **The Electrocardiogram and Cardiac Arrhythmias in Adults**

LABELING

1. On the illustration below, label the following: 0°, −30°, +30°, −60°, + 60, −90°, +90°, −120°, +120°, −150°, +150°, +180°, aV_R, aV_L, and aV_F, lead I, lead II, lead III, and the normal cardiac vector.

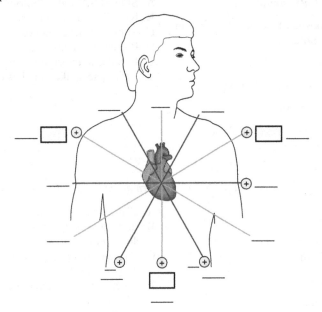

SHORT ANSWER/CRITICAL THINKING QUESTIONS

1. Draw an ECG waveform representing depolarization and repolarization. Label your diagram with the following: the P, Q, R, S, and T waves, the P-R interval and Q-T intervals, the ST segment, and the J point. Identify where atrial depolarization, ventricular depolarization, and ventricular repolarization occur.

2. Define the following terms:
   A. Lead (as it refers to electrocardiography)

B. Lead axis (for bipolar and unipolar leads)

C. Mean cardiac vector

3. Complete the following sentence: ECG graph paper contains small squares separated by light vertical lines that

are _____ mm apart, representing _____ second. Heavy vertical lines are _____ mm apart and represent

_____ second. Thus, there are _____ small squares between two heavy vertical lines. Five large squares

represent _____ second, and are _____ cm long. Thus, _____ inch of horizontal distance equals _____

second on ECG graph paper. The most common ECG recording time used for analysis is the _____ second strip,

with vertical "time" markers recorded every _____ seconds.

4. What determines whether a wave or complex recorded on the ECG will be deflected upward (positive) or downward
   (negative)?

5. Name all ECG leads and indicate whether they are bipolar or unipolar.

6. How is the hexaxial reference system constructed, and what is its purpose?

7. Using the hexaxial reference system, explain the location of the mean cardiac vector (MCV). Which "lead" runs parallel to the MCV? Will the QRS complex be positive or negative in this lead?

8. Fill in the blanks to complete the following sentence: If the QRS in lead I has an upward deflection, and the QRS in lead aV_F shows a downward deflection, then the mean direction of current flow during cardiac depolarization is

   between _____ degrees and _____ degrees, which represents a _____ axis deviation.

9. An ECG on a morbidly obese patient with severe COPD demonstrates a MCV of +150 degrees. How would you classify this electrical axis deviation? What could be causing this to occur?

10. What heart rates are associated with *tachycardia* and *bradycardia*?

11. Describe four steps used in ECG analysis.

12. A P-R interval greater than 0.2 seconds is indicative of what kind of electrical abnormality in the heart?

13. What causes a premature atrial contraction (PAC)? How is a PAC identified on ECG?

14. Why are the QRS complexes regular in atrial flutter but irregular in atrial fibrillation?

15. What is the cause of a *pulse deficit,* and which cardiac arrhythmia is associated with the development of it?

16. Differentiate the electrical abnormalities causing unifocal PVCs and multifocal PVCs. Which is the most dangerous pathology and why?

Chapter **19** **The Electrocardiogram and Cardiac Arrhythmias in Adults**

17. What conditions predispose the heart to ventricular fibrillation?

18. Differentiate the electrical abnormalities found in first, second, and third degree heart block.

CASE STUDIES

1. You are a respiratory therapist caring for a patient just admitted to the intensive care unit. This 84-year-old man was admitted for unexplained syncope (fainting) and hypotension. This patient's current weight is 81 kilograms (his normal weight) and he has a blood pressure of 85/48. The patient has been previously diagnosed with "mild" congestive heart failure. Now, an ECG reveals normal QRS complexes with a very irregular rhythm. No P waves are present on the ECG, but QRS complexes are connected by a fine, irregular baseline. The ventricular rate is approximately 160 beats per minute. Based on the patient's history and present findings, what is your conclusion about this patient's condition? What therapy is indicated?

2. You are called to the medical floor to administer a bronchodilator to a 28-year-old asthmatic patient complaining of increased respiratory distress and chest discomfort. An ECG was completed prior to your arrival and reveals the following: normal P, QRS, and T waves; regular rhythm; rate of 148 bpm. A pulse oximeter reading demonstrates an oxygen saturation of 88% on 2 L/min of supplemental oxygen, and the patient's peak flow readings are reduced 50% below her personal best. The patient's weight is stable and she has no history of heart disease, but she has been hospitalized twice in the past 2 years for acute exacerbations of asthma. What is your conclusion about this patient's condition? What therapy is indicated?

Using the four steps in electrocardiogram analysis found in Chapter 19, identify the arrhythmias associated with the following ECG tracings.

1.

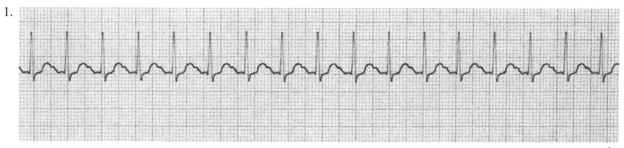

Lead II

2.

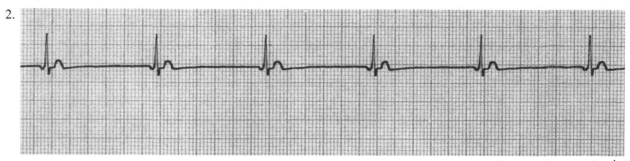

Lead II

3.

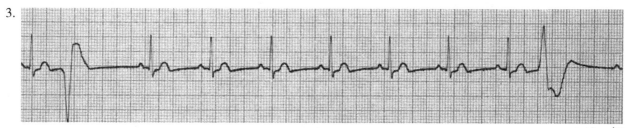

Lead II

4.

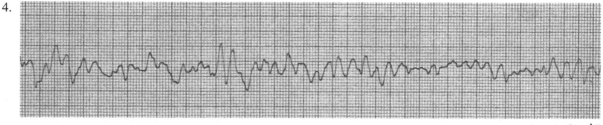

Lead II

(All ECG tracings from Seidel JC, editor: Basic electrocardiography: *a modular approach,* St. Louis, 1986, Mosby.)

20 Control of Cardiac Output and Hemodynamics

OBJECTIVES

After reading this chapter, you will be able to:

- Describe how various physiologic factors affect preload, afterload, and contractility.
- Distinguish between factors that affect venous return and factors that affect cardiac output.
- Identify the way in which cardiac output and venous return are interdependent.
- Use combined cardiac and venous return curves to illustrate the compensatory interaction between the heart and vasculature during abnormal hemodynamic conditions.
- Identify why decreased left ventricular contractility leads to pulmonary edema.
- Explain why various clinical hemodynamic measurements are indicators of preload, afterload, and contractility.
- Develop diagnostic classifications based on analysis of hemodynamic data.
- Develop a general therapeutic approach based on analysis of hemodynamic data.

KEY TERMS AND DEFINITIONS

Define the following terms:

1. Preload

2. Afterload

3. Contractility

4. Inotropic factors

5. Ejection fraction

6. Stroke volume

7. Mean circulatory filling pressure

8. Guyton diagram

9. Hemodynamic

10. Percutaneous catheterization

11. Pulmonary capillary wedge pressure (PCWP)

12. Pulmonary artery end-diastolic pressure (PAEDP)

13. Cardiac output

14. Cardiac index

15. Stroke volume index

16. Systemic vascular resistance index (SVRI)

17. Pulmonary vascular resistance index (PVR)

18. Left/right ventricular stroke work index (LVSWI or RVSWI)

19. Capillary hydrostatic pressure

20. Ventricular function curve

MATCHING

Hemodynamic Measurements

Match the normal range value on the right to the correct hemodynamic parameter on the left.

_____ 1. Cardiac output (CO)

_____ 2. Arterial blood pressure (BP)

_____ 3. Systemic vascular resistance (SVR)

_____ 4. Right atrial (central venous) pressure (RAP, CVP)

_____ 5. Pulmonary vascular resistance (PVR)

_____ 6. Pulmonary capillary wedge pressure (PCWP)

_____ 7. Mean arterial pressure (MAP)

_____ 8. Cardiac index (CI)

_____ 9. Stroke volume (SV) dynes•sec•cm^{-5}

_____ 10. Pulmonary artery pressure (PAP)

_____ 11. Heart rate (HR)

_____ 12. Left ventricular stroke work index (LVSWI)

_____ 13. Right ventricular stroke work index (RVSWI) dynes•sec•cm^{-5}

A. 60-130 mL/beat
B. 20-30/6-15 mm Hg
C. 2.5-4.0 L/min/m^2
D. 60-80 beats/min
E. 4-8 g-m/m^2/beat
F. Less than 6 mm Hg
G. 120/80 mm Hg
H. 4-8 L/min
I. 900-1400 dynes•sec•cm^{-5}
J. 4-12 mm Hg
K. 80-100 mm Hg
L. 40-75 g-m/m^2/beat
M. 100-250 dynes•sec•cm^{-5}

Hemodynamic Effects of Cardiovascular Drugs

Match the correct class of cardiovascular drug on the right to the appropriate therapeutic objective on the left.

_____ 1. Increase afterload

_____ 2. Increase contractility

_____ 3. Decrease preload

_____ 4. Decrease afterload

_____ 5. Increase preload

_____ 6. Decrease contractility

A. Vasodilator agents
B. Diuretic agents
C. Inotropic agents
D. Vasopressor agents
E. Negative inotropic agents
F. Intravenous fluids/blood transfusions

FILL IN THE BLANK

Provide the formulas used to calculate the following hemodynamic variables.

1. Cardiac index (CI) _____

2. Stroke volume (SV) _____

3. Stroke index (SI) _____

4. Systemic vascular resistance (SVR) _____

5. Pulmonary vascular resistance (PVR) _____

6. Left ventricular stroke work index (LVSWI) _____

7. Right ventricular stroke work index (RVSWI) _____

LABELING

1. Draw a Frank-Starling cardiac function curve, and place the correct label on each axis. Draw curves denoting normal, increased, and decreased contractility.

2. A. On the figure below, draw the pressure waveforms associated with location of the pulmonary artery catheter as is floated into position.

Chapter **20**   **Control of Cardiac Output and Hemodynamics**

B. Fill in the blanks with the normal pressures associated with each position of the pulmonary artery catheter.

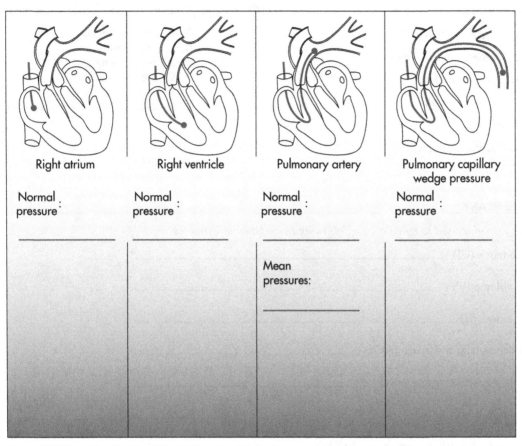

Right atrium

Normal
pressure

_____

Right ventricle

Normal
pressure

_____

Pulmonary artery

Normal
pressure

_____

Mean
pressures:

_____

Pulmonary capillary
wedge pressure

Normal
pressure

_____

(From Wilkins RL, Sheldon RL, Krider SJ: *Clinical assessment in respiratory care,* ed 3,
St Louis, 1995, Mosby.)

3. Write each of the following hemodynamic conditions in the appropriate quadrant of Forrester's hemodynamic subsets: normal hemodynamic state, acute left heart failure, fluid overload, dehydration, septic shock, and myocardial infarction.

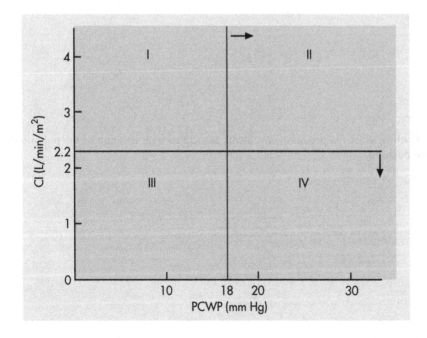

1. In what way does a high level of PEEP affect cardiac output, and why?

2. Why does left ventricular failure cause abnormally high PCWP and pulmonary edema? In what situation could pulmonary edema exist without a high PCWP?

3. What is the mechanism behind the abnormally high cardiac outputs seen in patients with septic shock?

4. How do calcium channel blocking drugs work to reduce myocardial oxygen consumption?

5. Which of the following pulmonary artery measurements may be elevated in the presence of observable jugular venous distention (JVD): CVP, MPAP, PCWP, PAP?

6. Describe the following about the pulmonary artery catheter:
   A. Measurement(s) obtained from each of the following: proximal lumen, distal lumen, thermistor

   B. The purpose of the balloon located near the distal lumen

   C. Significance of the dicrotic notch AND absence of the dicrotic notch on the pulmonary artery waveform

   D. Port from which a mixed venous blood sample would be drawn

7. Identify which hemodynamic measurement represents each of the following:
   A. Preload of the right ventricle

   B. Preload of the left ventricle

C. Afterload of the right ventricle

D. Afterload of the left ventricle

E. Contractility of the right ventricle

F. Contractility of the left ventricle

8. Describe the hemodynamic similarities and differences between hemorrhagic and cardiogenic causes of decreased cardiac output.

9. Compare the short- and long-term compensatory responses of the body to loss of myocardial contractility and why these responses may be both beneficial and harmful.

10. How can mechanical ventilation with PEEP therapy affect the interpretation of the PCWP?

CASE STUDIES

1. You are caring for a patient in the intensive care unit who has a history of chronic obstructive pulmonary disease with chronic hypoxemia. A pulmonary artery catheter has been placed to monitor the patient's hemodynamic status. Current measurements from the catheter include: CVP = 12 mm Hg, PAP = 40/20 mm Hg, PCWP = 16 mm Hg, and cardiac output and LVSWI are below normal. The patient's fluid status is verified as adequate by lab results and daily weights. The intensivist chooses to start an IV infusion of dopamine. (See Table 20-5 in text.)

   A. How does dopamine work?

   B. How will this patient's hemodynamic status be improved by the administration of dopamine?

174

C. What is the disadvantage of the drug for this type of patient? Dopamine has been administered and a new set of hemodynamic values include: CVP = 5 mm Hg, PAP = 45/15 mm Hg, PCWP = 10 mm Hg, cardiac output and LVSWI are within normal limits. Taking the patient's medical history into account:

D. Why is the systolic PAP value still abnormal?

E. Comment on the effectiveness of the inotropic drug.

2. A 58-year-old female with spinal cord injury has been hospitalized for several weeks. She is able to breathe without mechanical assistance. Past medical history includes treatment for angina and mild left ventricular failure. She suddenly develops severe chest pain, dyspnea, and tachypnea. She is immediately placed on oxygen via nasal cannula at 4 lpm and transported to the intensive care unit. A pulmonary artery catheter is placed and yields the following values:

Pulmonary Artery Catheter	ABGs	Vital Signs
CVP = 16 mm Hg	PO_2 = 80 mm Hg	HR = 130/min
PAP = 48/28	PCO_2 = 39 mm Hg	BP = 110/90 mm Hg
MPAP = 35 mm Hg	pH = 7.38	RR = 32/min
PCWP = 13 mm Hg	SaO_2 = .94	V_E = 12.8 L/min
CO = 4.5 L/min	Hb = 12 g/dL	MAP = 97 mm Hg
BSA = 1.7 m2		

Chapter 20 **Control of Cardiac Output and Hemodynamics**

A. What is your initial diagnostic impression, and which information supports your impression?

B. How do you explain the difference between the PA diastolic and PCWP?

C. Calculate the PVR, SVR, and CI, and state your final impression.

KEY CONCEPT QUESTIONS

*Instructions: Choose the **single** best answer for each multiple choice question.*

1. Right ventricular afterload is reflected by:
   A. Systemic vascular resistance
   B. Right atrial pressure
   C. Pulmonary capillary wedge pressure
   D. Pulmonary vascular resistance

2. Which of the following represents an immediate compensatory response to acute heart pumping failure:
   A. Sympathetic stimulation
   B. Decreased heart rate
   C. Systemic vasodilation
   D. Increased urine output

3. Pulmonary capillary wedge pressure (PCWP) is a reflection of:
   A. Right atrial pressure
   B. Right ventricular end-diastolic pressure
   C. Pulmonary vascular resistance
   D. Left atrial pressure

4. An abnormally high PCWP in a patient with a cardiac index of 3.5 and no valvular disease will be due to:
   A. High left ventricular stroke volume
   B. Low systemic vascular resistance
   C. High blood volume
   D. Low blood volume

176

21 Filtration, Urine Formation, and Fluid Regulation

OBJECTIVES

After reading this chapter, you will be able to:

- Identify the anatomy of the nephron.
- Differentiate between the terms filtrate and urine; reabsorption and secretion.
- Explain how glomerular filtration rate and urine output are related.
- Explain how autoregulation of the glomerular filtration rate and renal blood flow are related.
- Identify how the nephron processes the tubular filtrate to excrete a concentrated or dilute urine.
- Describe why it is important that the kidney's countercurrent multiplier mechanism maintains a high osmotic pressure deep in the medulla.
- Explain how aldosterone, natriuretic peptides, and antidiuretic hormone influence extracellular fluid volume.
- Identify the mechanisms whereby various classes of diuretic drugs work.

KEY TERMS AND DEFINITIONS

Define the following terms:

1. Afferent arteriole

2. Aldosterone

3. Angiotension

4. Antidiuretic hormone (ADH)

5. Atrial natriuretic hormone (ANH)

6. Bowman's capsule

7. Collecting duct

8. Cortex

9. Efferent arteriole

10. Filtration fraction

11. Glomerulus

12. Isotonic

13. Juxtaglomerular apparatus

14. Loop of Henle

15. Macula densa

16. Medulla

17. Nephron

18. Osmotic pressure

19. Peritubular capillaries

20. Renal corpuscle

21. Renin

22. Tubular transport maximum (Tm)

23. Vasa recta

MATCHING

Match the description to the correct term.

_____ 1. Point at which the filtrate becomes more concentrated

_____ 2. Place where 20% of the capillary blood's plasma is filtered

_____ 3. Actively pumps sodium ions out of the filtrate into the interstitial fluid

_____ 4. Point at which approximately 65% of the filtrate volume is absorbed

_____ 5. Responsible for the reabsorption of sodium and water to restore intravascular volume toward normal

_____ 6. Participates in the regulation electrolyte and fluid balance through reabsorption sodium and water in the presence of ADH

A. Ascending loop of Henle
B. Distal tubule
C. Bowman's capsule
D. Proximal tubule
E. Collecting duct
F. Descending loop of Henle

LABELING

1. Name each component of the nephron and trace blood flow and filtrate flow through the nephron.

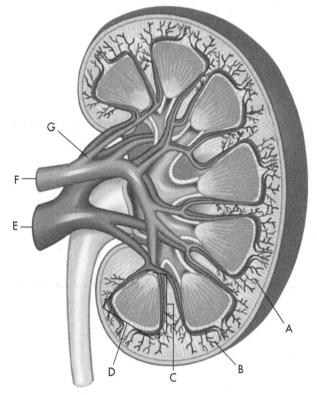

(From Patton KT, Thibodeau GA: *Anatomy & physiology,* ed 7, St. Louis, 2010, Mosby.)

A. _____

B. _____

C. _____

D. _____

E. _____

F. _____

G. _____

2. Number the following structures the glomerular filtrate flows through in the nephron after entering juxtamedullary nephron tubules, and explain what occurs in each structure.

_____ Loop of Henle

_____ Distal tubule

_____ Bowman's capsule

_____ Juxtaglomerular apparatus

_____ Proximal tubule

_____ Collecting duct

SHORT ANSWER/CRITICAL THINKING QUESTIONS

1. In addition to waste elimination and excretion, what other important roles do the kidneys play in the body?

2. Compare glomerular capillary blood pressure with pressures in the body's other capillary beds.

3. What effect does efferent arteriole constriction have on glomerular filtration rate (GFR)? Explain.

4. A. Compare the daily volume of substances filtered by the kidneys' glomeruli with the volume of substances ultimately excreted as urine.

B. What happens to this filtered volume?

5. Why is the osmotic pressure of the blood in the efferent arteriole so much different than the osmotic pressure in the afferent arteriole? (In your answer, note which has the higher osmotic pressure.)

6. Explain how the body keeps GFR fairly constant in the face of large blood pressure changes. Why is this important?

7. Differentiate the meaning of the terms *threshold* and *non-threshold* substances.

Chapter **21** **Filtration, Urine Formation, and Fluid Regulation**

8. The concentration of electrolytes (osmotic pressure) in the extracellular fluid surrounding the nephron tubules increases greatly from the cortex-medulla boundary to the bottom of the loop of Henle, deep in the medulla.
   (A) What factors contribute to this increased osmotic pressure at the bottom of Henle's loop? (Examine the following figures).

   (B) What is the purpose of maintaining the high osmotic pressure gradient described in (A) above? (How does this make it possible for the kidney to perform its intended function?)

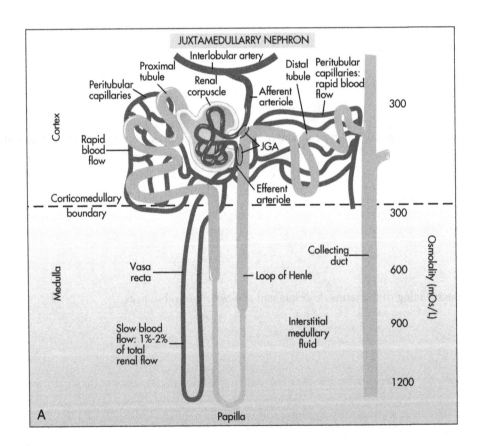

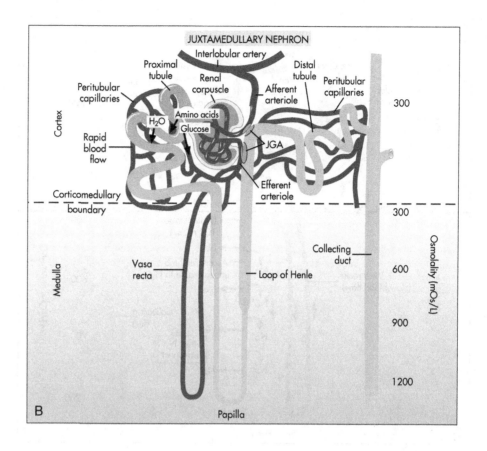

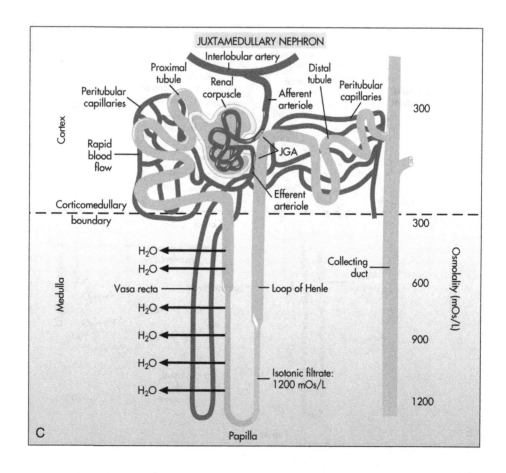

Chapter **21** **Filtration, Urine Formation, and Fluid Regulation**

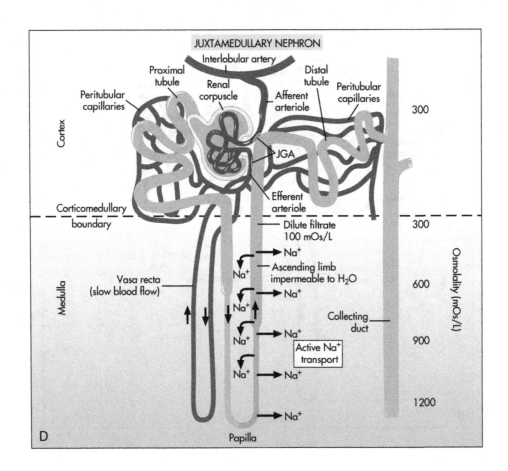

JUXTAMEDULLARY NEPHRON

Interlobular artery

Proximal tubule

Renal corpuscle

Distal tubule

Peritubular capillaries

Afferent arteriole

Peritubular capillaries

JGA

Efferent arteriole

Cortex

Corticomedullary boundary

Dilute filtrate 100 mOs/L

Na⁺

Na⁺

Ascending limb impermeable to H₂O

Vasa recta (slow blood flow)

Na⁺

Na⁺

Medulla

Na⁺

Na⁺

Collecting duct

Na⁺

Na⁺

Active Na⁺ transport

Na⁺

Na⁺

Na⁺

300

300

Osmolality (mOs/L)

600

900

1200

D

Papilla

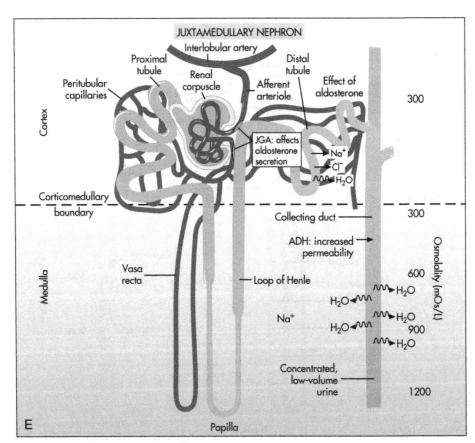

JUXTAMEDULLARY NEPHRON

Interlobular artery

Proximal tubule

Renal corpuscle

Distal tubule

Peritubular capillaries

Afferent arteriole

Effect of aldosterone

300

Cortex

JGA: affects aldosterone secretion

Na⁺

Cl⁻

H₂O

Corticomedullary boundary

Collecting duct

300

ADH: increased permeability

Vasa recta

Loop of Henle

600

H₂O

H₂O

Na⁺

Medulla

H₂O

H₂O

900

H₂O

Concentrated, low-volume urine

1200

Osmolality (mOs/L)

E

Papilla

9. Explain what causes the body to secrete aldosterone, or antidiuretic hormone (ADH), or atrial natriuretic hormone (ANH), and explain the role of these hormones in regulating the body's fluid volume.

10. A very common powerful "loop" diuretic is Lasix (furosemide). Explain how Lasix causes diuresis.

CASE STUDY

1. A 65-year-old male presents to the emergency room with complaints of increasing shortness of breath, orthopnea (dyspnea while lying flat), and fatigue. The patient has a history of hypertension and is recovering from a myocardial infarction he suffered 4 months ago. Physical exam reveals the following:

BP = 100/60 mm Hg
HR = 93 beats/min
RR = 22 breaths/min
Temp = 37° C
Weight = 93 kg (up 4 kg in the past week)
Breath sounds = crackles throughout both lungs
Swelling of the ankles (pedal edema)

A chest x-ray examination shows evidence of cardiomegaly and pulmonary edema. A diagnosis of congestive heart failure is made and the patient is started on furosemide (Lasix).

A. What is the mechanism by which the kidneys in a patient with congestive heart failure would actually *increase* water retention?

B. What is the rationale for starting Lasix? Explain the mode of action of this drug.

Chapter **21** **Filtration, Urine Formation, and Fluid Regulation**

C. What are some complications that might occur with the use of Lasix? Explain.

KEY CONCEPT QUESTIONS

*Instructions: Choose the **single** best answer for each multiple choice question.*

1. What percentage of the cardiac output flows through the kidneys?
   A. 100%
   B. 60%
   C. 40%
   D. 20%

2. The nephron reabsorbs all of the following *except*:
   A. Water
   B. Creatinine
   C. Electrolytes
   D. Glucose

3. Total urine output is approximately:
   A. 700 mL
   B. 100 mL
   C. 1500 mL
   D. 2000 mL

4. Urine volume is increased by the increased secretion of:
   A. Renin
   B. Atrial natriuretic hormone
   C. Aldosterone
   D. Antidiuretic hormone

Electrolyte and Acid-Base Regulation

KEY TERMS AND DEFINITIONS

Define the following terms:

1. Ammonia buffer system

2. Blood urea nitrogen

3. Chronic renal failure

4. Cotransport

5. Countertransport

6. Glomerulonephritis

7. Nephrotic syndrome

8. Phosphate buffer system

9. Postrenal failure

10. Primary active transport

11. Secondary active transport

12. Sodium-potassium-adenosine triphosphate pump

13. Uremia

LABELING

Label and draw arrows on the illustration below to represent the following:

A. Hypokalemia leading to alkalemia
B. Alkalemia leading to hypokalemia
C. Acidemia leading to hyperkalemia
D. Hyperkalemia leading to acidemia

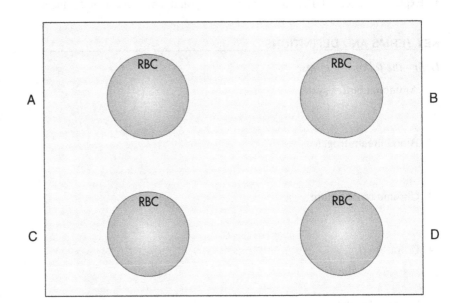

SHORT ANSWER/CRITICAL THINKING QUESTIONS

1. Describe the general importance of the buffers (base) in the filtrate. (For example, what would happen if they were not present?)

Chapter **22** **Electrolyte and Acid-Base Regulation**

2. Explain specifically what causes the tubules to secrete ammonia into the filtrate and how this helps the kidney do its work.

3. Explain the kidney's response to both respiratory acidosis and respiratory alkalosis. (Discuss each event, and show how the entire process restores blood pH back to the normal range.)

4. Explain why ammonia secretion is most extensive in people with COPD who have chronically high PaCO$_2$ and how this leads to hypochloremia in these people.

5. Explain how the lack of chloride ions leads to alkalemia and hypokalemia.

6. Explain how hypokalemia causes events that lead to "metabolic" alkalemia.

7. Which represents the most severe potassium depletion:
   A. Hypokalemia coexisting with alkalemia, or
   B. Hypokalemia coexisting with acidemia? Explain.

8. Why does severe dehydration lead to alkalemia?

CASE STUDY

1. A 74-year-old male is admitted to the hospital for pneumonia. The patient has a history of COPD and chronic CO_2 retention. Bronchodilator therapy and aggressive bronchial hygiene were started; however, the patient's respiratory status is showing signs of deterioration. His respiratory rate has increased from 22 breaths/min to 30 breaths/min and his SpO_2 has decreased to 85% on 2 L/min NC. Lab results reveal an elevated white blood count (consistent with pneumonia), elevated total CO_2 (consistent with chronic hypercapnia), and elevated blood urea nitrogen (BUN) and creatinine (Cr). An arterial blood gas (ABG) is ordered.

   A. What is the significance of the elevated BUN and Cr levels?

   B. Why is an ABG needed?

C. What do you expect the ABG to reveal?

KEY CONCEPT QUESTIONS

Instructions: Choose the **single** best answer for each multiple choice question.

1. The body places the highest priority on maintaining normal concentration of:
   A. Potassium
   B. Sodium
   C. Chloride
   D. Bicarbonate

2. In primary active transport, the ions that are normally transported from the blood into the tubular epithelial cells are the:
   A. Hydrogen ions
   B. Chloride ions
   C. Potassium ions
   D. Bicarbonate ions

3. In the process of secondary active secretion of potassium and hydrogen ions:
   A. Hydrogen is transported into the tubular cell.
   B. Sodium diffuses into the tubular cell.
   C. Potassium diffuses into the tubular cell.
   D. Chloride is transported into the tubular cell.

4. In most tubular segments, which ion is normally reabsorbed with sodium?
   A. Chloride
   B. Bicarbonate
   C. Potassium
   D. Hydrogen

23 Cardiopulmonary Response to Exercise in Health and Disease

OBJECTIVES

After reading this chapter, you will be able to:

- Describe why continual regeneration of adenosine triphosphate is necessary to sustain exercise.
- Explain how aerobic and anaerobic metabolic processes differ in their ability to generate adenosine triphosphate.
- Explain how oxygen consumption and carbon dioxide production differ in aerobic metabolism of carbohydrates and fats.
- Identify why the changes in respiratory, cardiovascular, and metabolic processes are different below than above the anaerobic threshold.
- Explain how caloric expenditure is related to oxygen consumption.
- Utilize exercise test data to differentiate cardiac and pulmonary limitations to exercise.
- Understand why sedentary and athletically trained individuals differ in their ability to perform exercise.
- Utilize exercise test data to differentiate obstructive and restrictive pulmonary limitations to physical activity.
- Utilize exercise test data to prescribe appropriate physical activity in cardiopulmonary rehabilitation programs.

KEY TERMS AND DEFINITIONS

Define the following terms:

1. Adenosine triphosphate (ATP)

2. Aerobic

3. Anaerobic

4. Anaerobic glycolysis

5. Anaerobic threshold (AT)

6. Breathing reserve (BR)

7. Cardiac capacity

8. Glycogen

9. Heart rate reserve (HRR)

10. Indirect calorimetry

11. Isocapnic buffering

12. Maximum exercise ventilation ($\dot{V}_E$max)

13. Maximum heart rate (HR_{max})

14. Maximum oxygen consumption ($\dot{V}O_2$max)

15. Maximum voluntary ventilation (MVV)

16. Metabolic cart

17. Metabolic equivalent (MET)

18. Oxygen pulse (O_2 pulse)

19. Pyruvic acid

20. Respiratory exchange ratio (R)

21. Respiratory quotient (RQ) ($\dot{V}CO_2/\dot{V}O_2$)

22. Ventilatory equivalent for carbon dioxide ($\dot{V}_E/\dot{V}CO_2$)

23. Ventilatory equivalent for oxygen ($\dot{V}_E/\dot{V}O_2$)

24. V-slope method

TRUE OR FALSE

Differentiating Carbohydrate and Fat Metabolism

Identify each of the following statements as true (T) or false (F) regarding fat and carbohydrate (glucose) metabolism.

_____ Metabolism of fat requires more oxygen than metabolism of carbohydrates.

_____ Carbohydrate metabolism generates more carbon dioxide than fat metabolism.

_____ Fat cannot be metabolized anaerobically.

_____ Carbohydrate metabolism requires more ventilatory work than fat metabolism.

_____ The major source of energy during maximal exercise is carbohydrate metabolism.

_____ The respiratory quotient (RQ) is greater for carbohydrates than for fats.

FILL IN THE BLANK

Aerobic Versus Anaerobic Metabolism

Indicate whether each of the following statements identifies processes involved in aerobic metabolism (A) or anaerobic metabolism (AN) or both (B).

_____ 1. The majority of energy sources for exercise come from glucose metabolism.

_____ 2. Bicarbonate ions buffer lactic acid, generating more carbon dioxide.

_____ 3. Glucose breaks down into pyruvic acid.

_____ 4. One molecule of glucose produces 36 molecules of ATP.

_____ 5. Occurs in the presence of oxygen.

_____ 6. Occurs in the absence of oxygen.

_____ 7. One molecule of glucose produces two molecules of ATP.

_____ 8. Creatine phosphate breaks down.

Differentiating Cardiac and Pulmonary Causes of Exercise Intolerance

Indicate whether each of the following statements represents a cardiac (C) or pulmonary (P) cause of exercise intolerance.

_____ 1. Maximum heart rate reached at low work rate

_____ 2. Severe dyspnea due to limited diffusion capacity

_____ 3. MVV is reached while heart rate is below predicted maximum

_____ 4. Low O_2 pulse and $\dot{V}O_2$max

_____ 5. Abnormally high heart rate for a given cardiac output

_____ 6. Severe dyspnea due to poor cardiac output decreasing oxygen delivery to tissues

Chapter **23** **Cardiopulmonary Response to Exercise in Health and Disease**

_____ 7. Inability to increase minute ventilation to perform more work

_____ 8. Limited ability to increase stroke volume

_____ 9. Severe dyspnea due to limited ventilatory capacity

_____ 10. Higher resting minute ventilation combines with lower MVV to reduce BR

_____ 11. Anaerobic threshold reached at low work rate

MATCHING

Exercise Testing Terminology

All of the following terms refer to terminology used in exercise testing. Match the definitions below with the correct symbol or term.

_____ 1. $\dot{V}O_2max$ (Maximum oxygen consumption)

_____ 2. O_2 pulse (Oxygen pulse)

_____ 3. $\dot{V}_Emax$ (Maximum exercise ventilation)

_____ 4. $\dot{V}_E/\dot{V}CO_2$ (Ventilatory equivalent for carbon dioxide)

_____ 5. BR (Breathing reserve)

_____ 6. HR_{max} (Maximum heart rate)

_____ 7. R (Respiratory exchange ratio)

_____ 8. RQ (Respiratory quotient)

_____ 9. $\dot{V}_E/\dot{V}O_2$ (Ventilatory equivalent for oxygen)

_____ 10. MVV (Maximum voluntary ventilation)

_____ 11. HRR (Heart rate reserve)

_____ 12. MET (Metabolic equivalent)

A. Minute ventilation increases at a higher rate than CO_2 production
B. Amount of oxygen consumed per minute, per kilogram of body weight
C. Maximum capacity of the body to transport and utilize oxygen
D. Minute ventilation increases at a higher rate than oxygen consumption
E. Amount of oxygen consumed or delivered per heart beat
F. The difference between MVV and $\dot{V}_Emax$
G. The amount of air breathed in and out, with maximal effort, over 10 to 15 seconds
H. Maximum predicted heart rate per minute (220 – age in years)
I. The ratio between carbon dioxide elimination and oxygen uptake
J. The difference between predicted maximum heart rate and observed heart rate
K. The ratio of CO_2 molecules produced to O_2 molecules consumed by the tissues
L. Maximum ventilation attained during exercise

1. Complete the flow diagram below, identifying the effects of cardiac disease limitation on exercise tolerance.

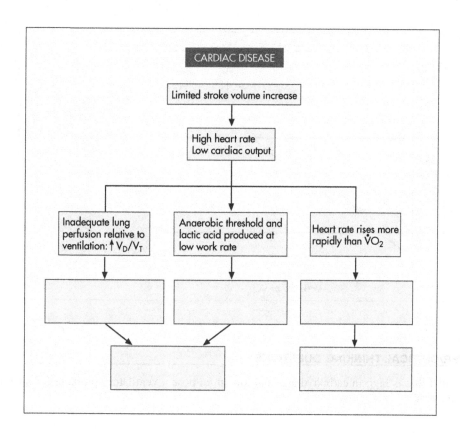

2. On the graph below:

   A. Draw a slope representing the work rate/$\dot{V}_E$ relationship for a patient with obstructive lung disease.

B. Identify the following: resting $\dot{V}_E$ for normal lungs, resting $\dot{V}_E$ for obstructive disease, MVV for normal lungs, MVV for obstructive disease, breathing reserve for normal lungs, breathing reserve for obstructive lung disease, maximum exercise $\dot{V}_E$ for normal lungs, maximal exercise $\dot{V}_E$ for obstructive lung disease.

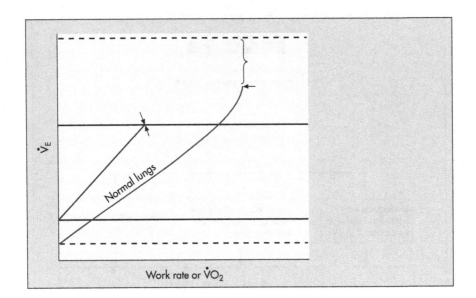

SHORT ANSWER/CRITICAL THINKING QUESTIONS

1. Why might a diet that is high in carbohydrates and low in fat pose a ventilatory problem for a COPD patient with chronic hypercapnia?

2. Why does an increased level of physical fitness decrease resting heart rate?

3. What is *cardiac capacity,* and how does it affect exercise performance?

4. As work rate increases, oxygen consumption increases. Why does the rate of oxygen consumption *decline* during exercise in the presence of cardiac disease?

5. Discuss each of the following in the context of an individual found to have a decreased ventricular ejection fraction:
   A. Time required to reach maximal exercise

   B. Heart rate reserve (HRR) at maximal exercise

   C. Oxygen pulse (O_2 pulse) and how it will compare to O_2 pulse in a healthy individual

6. In what way does the HRR of a patient with severe COPD differ from normal HRR, and why?

Chapter **23** **Cardiopulmonary Response to Exercise in Health and Disease**

7. What is meant by the term *oxygen debt*? How will pulmonary disease affect oxygen debt, ATP formation, and the pH of an individual performing exercise?

8. What physiologic abnormalities contribute to exercise limitation in individuals with pulmonary disease?

CASE STUDIES

1. A 70-year-old male has completed an exercise test, and you are asked to evaluate the test results. The patient's maximal heart rate was 150 beats/min and after reaching anaerobic threshold, $\dot{V}CO_2/\dot{V}O_2$ increased modestly; breathing reserve was 30% of MVV; and minute ventilation and carbon dioxide elimination increased more rapidly than oxygen consumption. Calculate the HRR for this patient, comment on all test results, and indicate whether the information given represents normal or abnormal test results.

2. Results from a patient's exercise test yield the following information: ventilatory reserve at maximum exercise was greater than normal; heart rate rose more rapidly than $\dot{V}O_2$ (low O_2 pulse); maximum heart rate and anaerobic threshold were reached at relatively low work rate; and the V_D/V_T ratio was high. Although the patient has no history of pulmonary disease, some of the test results are consistent with pulmonary limitation to exercise. Which test results could be indicative of pulmonary disease? Do the test results as a whole indicate pulmonary or cardiac exercise limitation?

*Instructions: Choose the **single** best answer for each multiple choice question.*

1. The normal primary limiting factor of exercise intensity in healthy individuals is:
   A. Stroke volume
   B. Cardiac capacity
   C. Maximum attainable minute ventilation
   D. V_D/V_T

2. In what way does the response to exercise differ in physically fit versus physically unfit people of the same age performing the same work?
   A. The maximum heart rates are lower in physically unfit people.
   B. Oxygen consumption is lower for the same work in physically fit people.
   C. Oxygen delivery rate is higher in physically unfit people.
   D. Cardiac output is higher at a given heart rate in physically fit people.

3. Compared to exercise test results of a patient with COPD, test results for a patient with restrictive lung disease are different because patients with restrictive lung disease have:
   A. Lower breathing reserves
   B. Low V_D/V_T
   C. Breathing rates > 50/min at maximum exercise
   D. Inadequate $\dot{V}_E$ response to lactic acidosis

4. People with severe obstructive airway disease are limited during exercise because:
   A. They reach maximum heart rate before their ventilation limit
   B. Their ability to eliminate CO_2 exceeds their ability to deliver O_2 to tissues
   C. They have above normal maximum voluntary ventilation
   D. They are unable to provide the minute ventilation required to do more work.

24 Effects of Aging on the Cardiopulmonary System

OBJECTIVES

After reading this chapter, you will be able to:

- Explain why health care of the elderly has taken on increasingly greater importance in the 21st century.
- Identify why older people are more prone to falls and how this phenomenon is related to pulmonary health.
- Identify why the elderly are more predisposed to infections than the younger population.
- Describe the nature of major age-related physiologic changes of the respiratory and cardiovascular systems.
- Describe the nature of the body's compensatory responses to age-related cardiopulmonary changes.
- Explain why the PaO_2 of the healthy elderly person is lower than that of the younger person when both individuals are breathing room air.
- Identify why the elderly person has a lower maximum cardiac output and oxygen consumption during exercise than the younger person.
- Explain the major benefits of an exercise program for the elderly individual.

KEY TERMS AND DEFINITIONS

1. baby boomers

2. kyphoscoliosis

3. senile emphysema

SHORT ANSWER/CRITICAL THINKING QUESTIONS

1. What *structural* changes occur in the respiratory system as a result of the aging process?

2. What *functional* changes occur in the respiratory system as a result of the aging process?

3. What clinical manifestations are associated with these changes?

4. What structural changes occur in the cardiovascular system as a result of the aging process?

5. What functional changes occur in the cardiovascular system as a result of the aging process?

6. What clinical findings are associated with these changes?

CASE STUDY

You are a respiratory therapist working in the emergency department when a 92-year-old man is brought in by ambulance. The patient's son witnessed the patient losing consciousness and falling to the ground after standing up to leave the table at the conclusion of their evening meal. The son reported that his father regained consciousness after the fall, but had a weak pulse and was unable to get up off the floor and into a chair. On admission, the patient is alert and oriented with the following vital signs: heart rate = 54 beats per minute, blood pressure = 100/64 mmHg, and he is breathing 14 times per minute. Assuming no underlying pathology is found, what functional changes associated with advanced age could have caused this man to lose consciousness and fall?

*Instructions: Choose the **single** best answer for each multiple choice question.*

1. Which of the following groups is growing the fastest, in both the United States and the world?
   A. Those aged 80 and older
   B. Those aged 85 and older
   C. Those aged 90 and older
   D. Those aged 95 and older

2. How does the lung function (in general) of a healthy 70-year-old compare to the lung function of a healthy 30-year-old?
   A. A 70-year-old has 80% of the lung function of a 30-year-old.
   B. A 70-year-old has 50% of the lung function of a 30-year-old.
   C. A 70-year-old has 30% of the lung function of a 30-year-old.
   D. A 70-year-old has 20% of the lung function of a 30-year-old.

3. Which of the following represents a normal, age-related change to the respiratory system:
   A. Decreased vital capacity
   B. Increased diffusion capacity
   C. Decreased residual volume
   D. Increased $PaCO_2$

4. Which of the following represents a normal age-related change to the cardiovascular system?
   A. Decreased vascular resistance
   B. Increased response to beta-adrenergic stimulation
   C. Decreased cardiac output
   D. Mitral valve regurgitation

Printed in the United States
By Bookmasters